A Time To Be Old, A Time To Flourish
The Special Needs of the Elderly-At-Risk

Report of
The Catholic Health Association's
Task Force on Long Term Care Policy

As Approved
by CHA Board of Trustees
June 20, 1988

The Catholic Health Association of the United States
St. Louis, MO

Photo on page 22 copyrighted by Roman Sapecki.

ISBN 0-87125-151-5

Table of Contents

FOREWORD

Few issues command greater attention or stir more emotions than our society's response to the special and often expensive needs of our rapidly growing elderly population. With older Americans as a group living much longer than ever before, people are increasingly concerned about how they and their relatives will be cared for should they become chronically ill.

This anxiety is naturally reflected in our nation's political life where candidates, legislators, and appointed officials are grappling with the difficult task of whether, and how best, to develop affordable, yet high quality and appropriate, programs of long term care. The effort is often marked by serious disagreements about the value of existing programs as well as the proper balance to be struck between public and private responsibility. Additionally, budget constraints cause some policymakers to wonder whether elderly Americans are already receiving too much in the way of care and services and to suggest that access by the elderly to some health and social services should be curtailed.

This report, *A Time To Be Old, A Time To Flourish: The Special Needs of the Elderly-At-Risk,* is The Catholic Health Association's attempt to inform rather than merely monitor this often confusing public policy debate. Even more importantly, it is an attempt to provide support and guidance to the Catholic healthcare ministry—whether manifested in hospitals, nursing homes, Charities agencies or parishes—as it attempts to discern its various ministerial responses to the frail elderly and their families. This report, then, recognizes that America's growing elderly population represents a challenge not just to society and government, but to the entire Church.

Fortunately, the Church in the United States has been generously blessed with substantial resources to help it respond to that challenge. Today's Catholics are the stewards of an institutional legacy of enormous value; the more than 1,000 Catholic healthcare facilities, the numerous Charities and home care agencies, the large number of colleges and universities, and the Church's nearly 18,000 parishes represent only a partial inventory of the rich array of resources available to the Catholic community. Understood within the context of our faith, they become a gift to be used creatively in the noble task of improving the lot of our fellow human beings, especially of the poor and the frail.

Thus, *A Time To Be Old, A Time To Flourish: The Special Needs of the Elderly-At-Risk* invites us to renew our sense of common purpose. Most of all, this report urges us to deepen our self-understanding as a *caring* community. A caring community embodies a number of characteristics, but the two most important are poverty and compassion.

Poverty is the inner understanding that our institutional heritage does not belong to us, nor is it property to be defended, accumulated, and strengthened for its own sake. Rather, it stands as an important but gentle reminder of our call to give, not only love and work, but life itself.

Compassion enables us to approach the frail elderly and their families not as the strong who pity the weak, but humbly and with the knowledge that together we can grow in our capacity to be more fully human. "This is what is demanded by the present moment and above all by the very dignity of the human person, the indestructible image of God the Creator, which is identical in each one of us" (*Sollicitudo Rei Socialis,* no. 47).

A Time To Be Old, A Time To Flourish: The Special Needs of the Elderly-At-Risk recognizes that the cultivation of these qualities in the daily operation of our healthcare institutions and services does not represent a simultaneous rejection of the principles of good business practice nor does it constitute evidence of managerial weakness. Rather, this report reflects a profound understanding of the purpose for which we continue to dedicate ourselves as ministry. Paradoxically, this report also is the source of the courage, energy, indeed, the confidence we will need to take the larger risks necessary to meet successfully the challenge to serve our frail elderly sisters and brothers.

In all of this, we are not alone, for as Pope John Paul II has recently reminded us,

> "[The Lord] unites us with himself and with one another by a bond stronger than any natural union, and thus united, he sends us into the whole world to bear witness through faith and works, to God's love, preparing the coming of his kingdom and anticipating it, though in the obscurity of the present time" (*Sollicitudo Rei Socialis,* no. 48).

John E. Curley, Jr.
President
The Catholic Health Association

Preface

In its social concern, the Church calls out to all people of good will on behalf of the victims of socio-economic injustice and the cultural and spiritual deprivation caused by it. "The joys and the hopes, the griefs and the anxieties of the people of this age, especially those who are poor or in any way afflicted, these too are the joys and hopes, the griefs and anxieties of the followers of Christ. Indeed, nothing genuinely human fails to raise an echo in their hearts" (*Gaudium et Spes,* no. 1). Today, this sense of human solidarity and social concern moves the Church to advocate on behalf of those elderly persons who are at risk in the United States, especially those who are poor.

In the absence of coherent public policy in the area of long term care and the admittedly uneven attempts of the private sector to meet their affective, cultural, and social needs, the elderly-at-risk face a labyrinth of uncertainty. The Church hears not only the echos of their need but the voice of the Lord himself: "When you saw me hungry or thirsty, a stranger or naked, sick or in prison, you came to help me" (Mt. 25:31-46).

The following report then, represents the Catholic healthcare ministry's reflection on the present need and perennial call. It is a further attempt to be true to our identity as servants and advocates for those who are vulnerable, while at the same time assuming a constructive role in a critical public discussion.

We expect our recommendations to be woven into the fabric of a much larger debate. It will take time to resolve the problems surrounding the care of the elderly-at-risk; but, as Pope John Paul II has counselled with regard to all social development: "This path is long and complex, and what is more it is constantly threatened because of the intrinsic frailty of human resolutions and achievements and because of the mutability of very unpredictable external circumstances. Nevertheless, one must have the courage to set out on this path and, where some steps have been taken or a part of the journey made, the courage to go on to the end." (*Sollicitudo Rei Socialis,* no. 38)

We have taken a first step and invite you to join with us in solidarity with the frail elderly to develop a consciousness in America of an aging society which offers a promise of opportunity to develop spiritually and a challenge to respond effectively.

Bishop Joseph M. Sullivan, DD
Auxiliary Bishop of Brooklyn
Chairman, CHA Task Force on
Long Term Care Policy

Acknowledgements

The Task Force wishes to thank and acknowledge the help of Sr. Elizabeth McMillan, RSM, PhD, Sr. Juliana Casey, IHM, PhD, Lawrence Seidl, and Laurence O'Connell, PhD, STD, of CHA's Division of Theology, Mission, and Ethics; Lola Westhoff, CHA Division of Member Services; Sr. Suzanne Sattler, IHM, Sisters of Mercy Health Corporation; Sr. Margaret Rose Whiteneck, CBS, Bon Secours Hospital–Villa Maria Nursing Center; Brother Joseph Berg, CSC, Catholic Charities USA; and James McCormack, PhD, Fordham University, in the preparation of this report. Special thanks also to Jeannie Moody, CHA Division of Government Services, for her unfailing patience in typing and retyping successive drafts of this document.

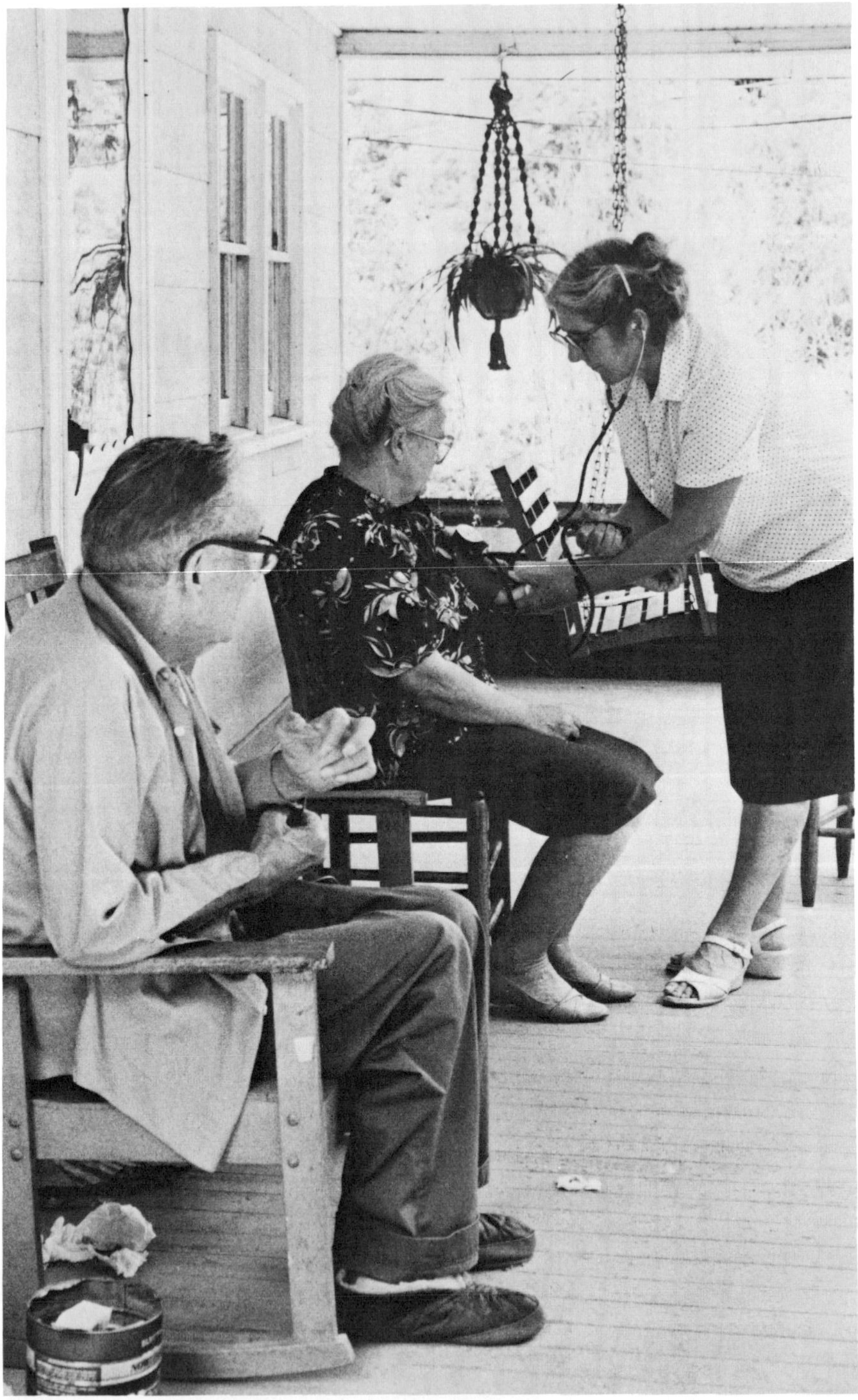

Introduction

In 1986, the Board of Trustees of The Catholic Health Association of the United States (CHA) established a select Task Force on Long Term Care Policy and charged it with a twofold purpose: to promote a better understanding of aging issues and their implications for the Church, its agencies, and social and public policy entities, and to call each of these groups to make additional, immediate, and long term commitments to help elderly persons who are at risk, especially those who are poor.

This document responds to that charge. It is a direct outgrowth of CHA's earlier study of the poor's healthcare needs, which resulted in the seminal report, *No Room in the Marketplace: The*

Health Care of the Poor.[1] That document focuses on the healthcare needs of all poor persons. Although it draws attention to the "plight of the elderly poor," its broad scope permits it to consider only briefly their problems and needs.

Task Force's Focus

This report's focus is the elderly-at-risk and their need for a coherent set of long term care services. It defines the elderly-at-risk as persons over 65 years of age who are presented with the reality or prospect of emotional, social, physical, mental, economic, environmental, or spiritual change that has reduced or might reduce their ability to live independently. These persons are often in need of informal or formal support to compensate them for their impairment. While there are other people (for example, chronically ill children and functionally impaired adults under 65) whose urgent long term care needs require similar study and recommendations, this Task Force's focus is the special needs of the frail elderly.

Urgent Initiative

This latest CHA initiative on long term care for the frail elderly is urgent for several reasons. *First,* the Catholic Church and its healthcare ministry exist in a society that is rapidly changing from a youthful to an older adult population. This reality has profound implications for healthcare service providers, other Church-related health ministries, families, and government as a growing number of older persons outlive their social, familial, and financial resources. This initiative is also a recognition that the phenomenon of a rapidly aging population is entirely new. Thus, our experience is limited, and we are not well prepared to meet this challenge.

The retired elderly population is now increasing more rapidly than the number of persons entering the work force. In 1985, the ratio was 19 elderly for every 100 people of working age, up from 7 per 100 in 1900. By the year 2020, the ratio is expected to rise to 29 per 100, and by 2050, 83 per 100. The reasons for this development are multiple: lower birthrates and extended life expectancy are the primary reasons, but it is also caused by the recent growth in early retirement, lower immigration (due to new immigration laws), and the AIDS epidemic, which is striking down large numbers of people in their most productive years.[2]

These trends indicate that increasing financial burdens are being placed on the working population to provide for the needs of the elderly and young persons. As Pope John Paul II has pointed out, this development forces us to ask the troubling question: "With what resources and in what forms will it be possible to promote and ensure an effective combination for real assistance to the elderly, so as to guarantee them a worthy and fitting lifestyle in keeping with their dignity and their affective, cultural and social needs, avoiding as far as possible anonymous and mass forms of assistance?"[3]

A *second* reason for serious concern is that our society is currently not doing as good a job as it should in meeting the needs of the frail elderly. As Chapter 1 makes clear, the nation's long term care policy is outmoded. Events are quickly outrunning the formulas of the past, placing severe burdens on many of the frail elderly and leaving the nation playing catch-up.

The fragmentation in funding for existing long term care services has tended to reinforce a fragmentation in service delivery. This has created a complex maze of programs that are often bewildering to the elderly-at-risk and their caregivers. Even when services are available, they are not always appropriate to the frail person's needs and preferences. It is difficult to not be troubled by the physical, financial, emotional, and social toll this nonsystem of long term care makes on people when they or their family members need care. This report calls for fundamental reform of our public and private long term care programs through the development of a coherent, rational, and integrated set of services focused on the frail elderly's functional needs. In Chapter 1, the Task Force suggests that this can best be conceptualized as a continuum of care.

A *third* and more disturbing worry is the recent development of a new and pernicious form of ageism that questions whether the elderly are still socially worthy recipients of governmental assistance. Proponents of this view argue that elderly poverty rates have dropped significantly and that the elderly are now in an economic position superior to that of the general population. They further maintain that the elderly already consume more than their "fair share" of society's resources. At the same time, they argue pressing unmet needs exist elsewhere in society; the growth in poverty rates among children is most frequently cited.

In this view, the elderly are no longer stereotyped as a primarily disabled, dependent, and vulnerable group, but as a "powerful political block enjoying benefits unavailable to any other age group, benefits that are no longer demonstrably needed and which are continued only at great cost to younger, working generations."[4] Some are even raising the specter of the imminent breakout of political intergenerational warfare.

This approach is little more than a contemporary form of ageism that replaces one set of derogatory images of the elderly with another set. It is also a politically and ethically dangerous prejudice. The underlying assumption of those appealing to this argument seems to be that monies realized from potential cutbacks in services to the elderly would automatically revert to children. This assumption is untenable considering the Reagan government's public policy priorities as expressed in higher defense budgets and lower domestic program spending and tax rates.

By focusing on the economic status of the elderly as a group, the argument also masks the fact that there are significant numbers of elderly who are still poor. In 1987, the U.S. Government "poverty line" for an elderly single person was $5,393 or $104 per week. Current estimates are that in 1987, 2.6 million elderly people were living in poverty.[5] Of the elderly individuals who live alone, poverty incidence is highest among minorities—43 percent for nonwhites and 35 percent for Hispanics, compared with 16 percent for whites.[6] Today, only 35 percent of elderly individuals who live alone have *any* pension income. Almost 70 percent of single older Americans will become impoverished within three months after entering a nursing home. Fifty percent of all couples are impoverished within six months after one spouse is admitted.[7] Furthermore, high out-of-pocket medical expenses for themselves or their husbands before death have impoverished many widows.

Contemporary ageism also tends to blind us to the fact that the elderly are financially better off as a group today precisely because of the existence of government programs such as Social Security and Medicare. Eliminate or significantly cut back such programs, and many more elderly would quickly become poor.

Finally, the modern stereotype of a vocal, voting senior citizen already enjoying unprecedented benefits politically impedes efforts to reform our current nonsystem of long term care into a more coherent and effective set of services that focuses on functional need. Therefore, it is important to note the obligation that organizations of the elderly have for exercising their considerable power responsibly.

As important as the preceding trends are to The Catholic Health Association's interest in long term care, an even more compelling motivation is supplied by our ministerial responsibility to do what we can to lighten the daily burdens borne by the frail elderly and their caregivers. The following true story adds an important human dimension to our analysis and helps us to better appreciate how considerable and unrelieved those burdens can sometimes be.

Ernestine's Story: A Personal Profile

"I have three problems," said the older woman. "I am old, sick, and poor." The woman's name is Ernestine, and she is 76 years old. She lives alone in a low-income neighborhood on $430 in monthly Social Security benefits, $44 worth of food stamps, and her wits.[8]

Once the resident manager of an apartment complex, Ernestine has a heart ailment, high blood pressure, and diabetes. She takes 10 different medicines each day. Her illnesses make it difficult for her to leave home, even to attend her church.

She says that she fears that she might lose her house to creditors as a result of a $1,000 medical bill she owes from her two heart attacks in 1986.

More than half of Ernestine's monthly Social Security check goes to her $239 monthly mortgage; the balance pays for electricity, heating, oil, telephone service, food, medicine, and minor home maintenance costs, such as repairing two porch steps. After those expenses are paid, Ernestine says, she has nothing left for medical costs that exceed her Medicare coverage.

Settled in a big stuffed chair in her living room, with her dog, Toy, bouncing and barking, she tries to make the best of her situation. The house is warm and tidy, soft music plays from a small radio, and a pile of crochet work, a telephone, and a stack of library books are nearby. This is Ernestine's world almost all the time.

"I haven't been out of the house in three months," she says. A friend picks up groceries and medicine for her and drops them off at her house. She receives a hot meal from the county five days a week as part of a program for the elderly. A caseworker with the county department of aging visits Ernestine or calls her regularly.

Nevertheless, Ernestine gets upset about the ups and downs of the benefit system on which she depends. When Social Security benefits rise as a result of the cost-of-living increase, she says, other benefits shrink, in part because of government formulas. For example, food stamp allotments are reduced when a recipient's income rises. Ernestine never seems to get ahead.

This month her Social Security check increased $12, from $418 to $430, because of a cost-of-living adjustment. At the same time, her monthly food stamp allowance dropped $8, from $52 to $44, the result of her higher Social Security check. Her net gain for the month is $4. "They give you with one hand," Ernestine says, "and take away with the other."

In the meantime, the hospital she was in during 1986, responding to a federal directive to try to collect unpaid bills, turned Ernestine's debt over to a collection agency. "They keep mailing me things, but I can't pay," she says, pulling out a letter from the agency. The most frightening development came, however, when the legal aid office told her to work out a payment plan with the hospital because her house could possibly be attached and sold by a creditor to satisfy bills that she owes. The county caseworker says that Ernestine is so emotionally attached to her home that "it would be her death" to have to move. "It's just a shack," says Ernestine, "but it's my shack."

Ernestine does not define all elderly-at-risk, but she typifies some of their characteristics and concerns. While the majority of the U.S. elderly are generally healthy and have sufficient incomes to live independently with little or no assistance, many like Ernestine do not.

Catholic Social Teaching

This report's response to the special needs of the frail elderly is anchored in Catholic social teaching. At the center of this teaching are the transcendence of God and the dignity of the human person. The human person is the clearest reflection of God's presence in the world; all the Church's work in pursuit of both justice and peace is designed to protect and promote the dignity of every person. Each person not only reflects God, but also is the expression of God's creative work and the meaning of Christ's redemptive ministry.

Therefore, the report is organized around a portrayal of the elderly-at-risk as persons of worth who have a place of respect and affection within the family, the home, the parish, the neighborhood, and the nation. The report reinforces the statement of Pope John Paul II that the elderly are "valuable resources of which the family (and society) can take advantage so as to avoid the impoverishment that results where these resources are ignored or forgotten."[9]

We believe that aging is not a reason for despair but a basis for hope, not a slow decaying but a gradual maturing, not a fate to be undergone but a chance to be embraced.

This discussion recognizes God's call to respond to the particular and varied needs of the frail elderly as a special opportunity for human and spiritual growth. It is an invitation that draws each of us beyond the elderly person's immediate needs and into a reflection in faith on the nature of aging, with the physical decline and dependence on others that are often associated with it. As the Bible reminds us, "Ask of your elders . . . let them enlighten you," (Dt 32:7).

Preferential Option for the Poor

The Church's recent social teachings articulate a "preferential option for the poor." This teaching reminds us that among the elderly-at-risk, the elderly poor are at greatest risk. Pope John Paul II has described the option for the poor as "a call to have a special openness with the small and weak, those that suffer and weep, those that are humiliated and left on the margins of society, so as to help them win their dignity as human persons and children of God."[10] This report focuses special attention on their needs. The 2.6 million elderly living in poverty are a silent constituency whose sheer number is a call to advocacy.

In this regard, the Task Force wishes to recognize that the U.S. Catholic Bishops have detailed three challenges to the contemporary Church that flow from such an option:

> "First, (the Contemporary Church) imposes a prophetic mandate to speak for those who have no one to speak for them, to be a defender of the defenseless who, in biblical terms, are the poor. It also demands a compassionate vision (Lk 10:33) which enables the Church to see things from the side of the poor, to assess lifestyle as well as social institutions and policies in terms of their impact on the poor. Finally and most radically, it calls for an emptying of self,

both individually and corporately, that allows the Church to experience the power of God in the midst of poverty and powerlessness."[11]

The preferential option for the poor implies a commitment to the revision of social structures. There is an ever-increasing concentration of wealth in the world. The preferential option calls for breaking up this concentration and developing a spirit of solidarity, both within and among nations. Redesigned economic structures must be put in place that guarantee each person in a society a reasonable share of certain basic or primary social goals.[12]

This report continues the CHA Stewardship Task Force emphasis on justice by using the term "service *of* the poor" rather than "service *to* the poor." That distinction serves to highlight the shift from a charity emphasis ("to the poor") to the justice intention that "the poor are served."[13]

Task Force Recommendations

This report will attempt to discern the responsibility of the whole Church, i.e., parishes and dioceses, state and national episcopal conferences (Chapter 3), Catholic healthcare providers (Chapter 4), and various levels of government (Chapter 5) for addressing the problems facing the elderly-at-risk. Chapter 5 also expresses the Task Force's strong support for a long term care social insurance program and examines the limited role of private long term care financing mechanisms. In each instance, the report makes a set of specific recommendations.

These recommendations are progressive and challenging. Consequently, many of them will be viewed as optimistic, perhaps even naive, considering the nation's current budget difficulties and the competitive and fiscal realities confronting healthcare organizations. Certainly, it would have been safer for the Task Force's recommendations to have lingered on the trailing edge of change than to surge ahead to the leading edge. The Task Force believes that by doing so, however, we in Catholic healthcare would lose the opportunity to continue moving toward our long-professed goal of placing the patient or client at the center of everything that we do.

In this regard, the Task Force wishes to emphasize an important point: long term care policy and this report are not primarily about the needs of facilities such as nursing homes and hospitals, or about programs, placements, cases, target groups, or "market opportunities"; their concern is frail elderly people and their families and communities—their lives. In the final analysis, long term care comes down to people caring for people. Whatever we may think of corporations, institutions, and governmental programs, the success of any reform in this area will depend on the availability of persons at every level who are motivated to help others. Successful reform will be measured by very small events in the lives of the frail elderly—"Is there someone there I can call? Do they make me feel like a person? Can I maintain my dignity and self-respect?" These are the issues by which all our actions on behalf of the frail elderly will be measured.[14]

In making its recommendations, this report regularly asks the question, "What is the best way to provide services to the elderly-person-at-risk?" The correct answer is often difficult to determine, but a careful and thoughtful effort to respond to it must be the departure point for any private or public program of care and any proposal for overall systemic change.

Although the policy goals and program recommendations in this report are compelling and demanding, the Task Force is not presenting them as the definitive and final word on the subject. The field of long term care is an evolving one. Thus, the Task Force hopes the reader will approach this report's analysis and recommendations as a helpful starting point for his or her own further reflection, discernment, and action.

At the outset of its report, the Task Force also wishes to draw all concerned parties' attention to the biblical admonition:

> O children, help your father and mother in their old age, and do not grieve them as long as they live; even if they are lacking in understanding, show forbearance; in all your strength do not despise them. For kindness to parents will not be forgotten, and against your sins it will be credited to you (Si 3:12-14).

NOTES

1. *No Room in the Marketplace: The Health Care of the Poor,* St. Louis, The Catholic Health Association of the United States, 1986.
2. Jack M. Guralnik, Dwight B. Brock, and Jacob A. Brody, "The Changing Demography of the Elderly in the United States," unpublished research paper, Bethesda, MD, National Institute on Aging, 1986.
3. Pope John Paul II, Address to the National Conference of the Italian Federation of Family Advisory Bureau of Christian Inspiration, March 28, 1987, *L'Osservatore Romano,* April 27, 1987, p. 12.
4. Bart J. Collopy, "Medicare: Ethical Issues in Public Policy for the Elderly," New York, Fordham University, September 1984. This paragraph and portions of the next several paragraphs in the text are based on arguments developed in this reference.
5. "Old, Alone and Poor: A Plan for Reducing Poverty Among Elderly People Living Alone," The Commonwealth Fund Commission on Elderly People Living Alone. Baltimore, 1987.
6. "Old, Alone and Poor," 1987.
7. "Nursing Home Care as a Work Benefit," *The Wall Street Journal,* June 30, 1988.
8. Molly Sinclair, "Living by Her Wits, and Not Much Else: 'Old, Sick, and Poor' in Prince George's," *Washington Post,* Jan. 18, 1988, p. B1.
9. Pope John Paul II.
10. Pope John Paul II, Address to Bishops of Brazil, 6.9, 10:9, July 31, 1980, p. 135.
11. "Catholic Social Teachings and the U.S. Economy," no. 51, *Origins* 14:22/23, Nov. 15, 1984, p. 346.
12. John F. Monagle and David C. Thomasma, eds., *Medical Ethics—A Guide for Health Professionals,* Rockville, MD, Aspen Publishers, 1988, p. 309.

13. “Stewardship Task Force Summation Report,” submitted to the CHA Board of Trustees, April 1984, St. Louis, The Catholic Health Association of the United States.
14. This insight into the matter of long term care is adapted from Rosalie A. Kane and Robert L. Kane, *Long-Term Care: Principles, Programs, and Policies,* New York, Springer Publishing Co., 1987, p. 383.

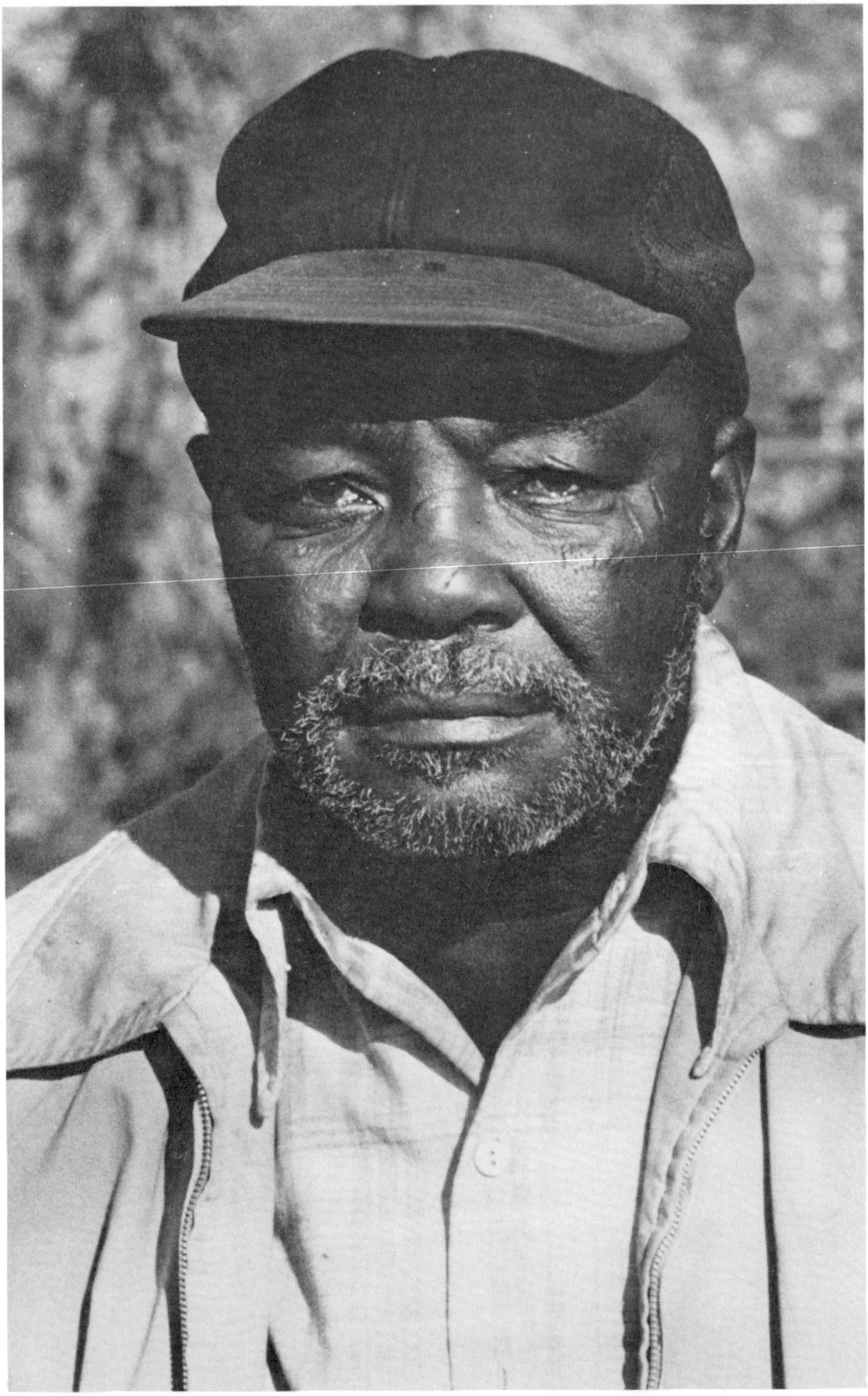

1

Elderly-At-Risk and Long Term Care

Americans over 65: A Demographic Profile

The number of persons similar to Ernestine (see Introduction) will grow as the elderly population increases dramatically in the United States, both in total numbers and as a percentage of the overall population. For the most part, this trend is going to continue well into the next century.

U.S. Census Bureau figures drive home the dimensions of this new and growing reality:[1]

- Between 1900 and the present, there has been an eightfold increase in the number of those persons over the age of 65 and almost a tripling of their proportion of the population.
- The number of Americans 65

and over is expected to swell from 29 million today to more than 34 million, or 12 percent of the population, in 12 years and more than 65 million by the year 2050.
- In 1985, for the first time in American history, the number of those persons over the age of 65 exceeded the number under the age of 18.

The most significant change in the U.S. population, however, is in the old-old population. The percentage of the very elderly, i.e., persons aged 85 or more, is rising sharply and will continue doing so into the indefinite future. Consider the following:

- Those aged 75 to 84 will increase to 35 percent of the elderly by the year 2000.
- The fastest growing segment of the U.S. population comprises those who are 85 and older. This group has increased from about 5 percent of the aged in 1960 to 9 percent in 1980, and it will reach 15 percent by the year 2000.
- A substantial change also has occurred even within the age structure of this old-old population. Those 90 to 94, 95 to 99, and 100+ each have increased as a proportion of the elderly over 85, with the proportionate increase greatest for those oldest. Those 100+ have increased threefold and now represent 1 percent of the aged population, numbering 23,000.

Although the numbers may seem small, continued accumulation of very old will have an increasing impact on requirements for health and social services and government responsibilities, as persons outlive their social, familial, and financial resources.

Implications for Increased Dependency

Whether these large increases in the life expectancy of persons over age 65 will produce a correspondingly large increase in the number of the elderly who are functionally impaired is less clear. One theory holds that the very factors that have caused people to live longer will also reduce the amount and seriousness of poor health among the very old. Thus, the extra years will generally be healthy and productive.[2]

This optimistic view is rejected by others who have concluded that the improvements in life expectancy mean that more disabled persons will survive. Thus, the older population is likely to be more disabled, not less. The most likely scenario incorporates both points of view. Some disabled persons who would have died will survive, and many who survive will be healthier than their forebears.[3]

In any event, several studies have established a clear correlation between aging and an increase in functional dependency. The correlation is often measured in terms of basic activities of daily living (ADLs), such as bathing, dressing, eating, and locomotion. (See Table 1.)

TABLE 1

Percentage of Persons 65 Years of Age and Over Living in the Community with Functional Dependencies, by Age and Sex: 1982

	ADL (activities of daily living) Limitation Score*				
Age/Sex	**Only IADL (limited)**	**1 to 2 (mildly disabled)**	**3 to 4 (disabled)**	**5 to 6 (severely disabled)**	**Total**
65 to 74					
Male	4.2	3.4	1.7	2.4	11.7
Female	4.8	4.7	1.9	1.9	13.3
75 to 84					
Male	7.1	6.5	2.5	4.6	20.9
Female	8.5	10.3	4.3	4.4	27.6
85+					
Male	9.9	15.7	7.7	7.5	40.8
Female	10.3	18.2	7.9	11.8	48.2

Tabulations from the 1982 National Long Term Care Survey (NLTCS) prepared by the Center for Demographic Studies, Duke University. Reported by Soldo and Manton, 1985; Rosalie A. Kane and Robert L. Kane, *Long Term Care: Principles, Programs, and Policies,* New York, Springer Publishing Co., 1987.

The data demonstrate the high functional dependency rates of the old-old elderly. Three times as many persons aged 85+ report needs for ADL help as those aged 65 to 74.

*Needs assistance with the instrumental activities of daily living (IADLs): managing money, shopping, light housework, meal preparation, making a phone call, taking medication. The score is the sum of the number of activities of daily living (ADL) with which respondent requires assistance: eating, bathing, dressing, toileting, etc.

Also of increasing concern is the correlation between age and the incidence of dementia. Studies of various population groups have shown prevalence rates from 3 to 20 percent in persons aged 65 and over who are living in the community. The prevalence in those who are institutionalized is considerably higher. It is a reasonable estimate that in the year 2000, 4 million people may have Alzheimer's disease, the most common dementia in the United States.[4]

As individuals move into their eighth and ninth decades of life, the probability of decreased function and disability substantially rises. The 1982 National Long Term Care Survey reported that three times as many persons aged 85+ report needs for ADL help than do those aged 65 to 74. Thus, the number of individuals at risk, while only a small portion of those over age 65, is a relatively large segment at age 85.[5]

Causes of Frailty and Dependence

The causes of frailty and dependence are both remote and proximate, and both should be the object of personal and societal concern.

The remote causes of frailty are rooted in the physical and social environment, in a person's genetic makeup and lifestyle. The air, water, amount and type of nourishment, values, role models and significant others, and personal choices ranging from automobiles to food, tobacco, and alcohol can all contribute to dependency. In some frail elderly, one of these factors is dominant; in most, however, several are at work.

The proximate causes of dependency may be trauma or disease of a physical and/or emotional nature. Personal choices may or may not be a factor in the etiology of the disabling condition.

It is important to note that dependency is not set and determined for all time; rather, it can move in various directions. Although "stages" may be observed in some diseases causing dependency, the actual degree of a person's dependency is the result of a complex set of psychological, physical, social, economic, and other factors. Two persons with identical underlying difficulties may exhibit very different degrees of dependency.

Thus, dependency in the elderly often results from chronic conditions that gradually take their toll, either as individual diseases or, more likely, as part of a complex of health, social, economic, and environmental conditions that combine to make daily living impossible without the help of others. Studies have shown that the dependent elderly tend to have more pain and discomfort, experience greater limitation in daily living, spend more days in bed, and suffer more often from depression than other adults. Caring for them can be a difficult, draining, time-consuming, and costly affair. While as few as 5 percent of the population over 65 may be in a nursing home on any given day, another 10 percent, similarly disabled, are being cared for by family, friends, and neighbors. In the 85 and older group, 23 percent are institutionalized.[6] In addition, such longstanding disabilities as chronic mental illness and mental retardation can be exacerbated by advanced age. Often, elderly persons with these impairments find themselves left out of the healthcare system.

The Plight of the Elderly-At-Risk Who Are Poor

Despite the improved economic status of many elderly citizens, a disturbingly high percentage of them are poor. (See Figure 1.) In 1985, 26 percent of men and 56 percent of women over age 65 had incomes below $7,000.[7] Of the 27 million noninstitutionalized elderly persons in the United States, almost 9 million live alone; of these, approximately 2 million are poor. Elderly persons who live alone are about five times as likely to be poor as elderly couples. About 67 percent of the elderly poor living alone are widows, revealing one of the predominantly feminine faces of poverty in the United States. Many of these widows suffered a sharp decline in income following the retirement or death of their husbands. Not surprisingly, the loss of pension income combined with large medical and funeral expenses contributed most dramatically to the rapid deterioration of their financial situation.[8]

Although the remaining elderly population is expected to do well assuming economic growth over the next 30 years, poverty rates among older citizens living alone will show only marginal improvements. As a group, those over age 75 are expected to experience no economic gains. Again, whereas male poverty will drop sharply by the year 2000, women will experience little improvement. Almost two thirds of black women age 85 or older who live alone are poor. By the year 2020, poverty among elderly persons will almost exclusively be a problem of elderly women living alone. The deficit suffered by elderly women living alone is not only economic; they need emotional support and help with physical tasks. Half of the elderly living alone are over age 75, and almost half are in poor or only fair health; they spent over 15 percent of their income on healthcare in 1985, an average of $1,660 per person.[9]

It is also important to remember that even the economically secure elderly can be quickly impoverished by such catastrophic costs as a serious illness or the need to provide skilled nursing care for a spouse. This risk will be significantly reduced by the Medicare catastrophic health legislation recently signed into law. The relative well-being of most elderly persons also does not constitute evidence that programs such as Social Security payments and Medicare benefits for the aged have become superfluous. The economic progress of the elderly in the United States is largely attributable to these programs, and if they were scrapped or seriously curtailed, many persons would be deprived of necessities. Even the severely strained Medicaid program with its serious access problems has provided a measure of security for some of the elderly who needed and could not afford nursing home care.

FIGURE 1

Poverty Rates Among Various Sub-Groups of Elderly People, 1987

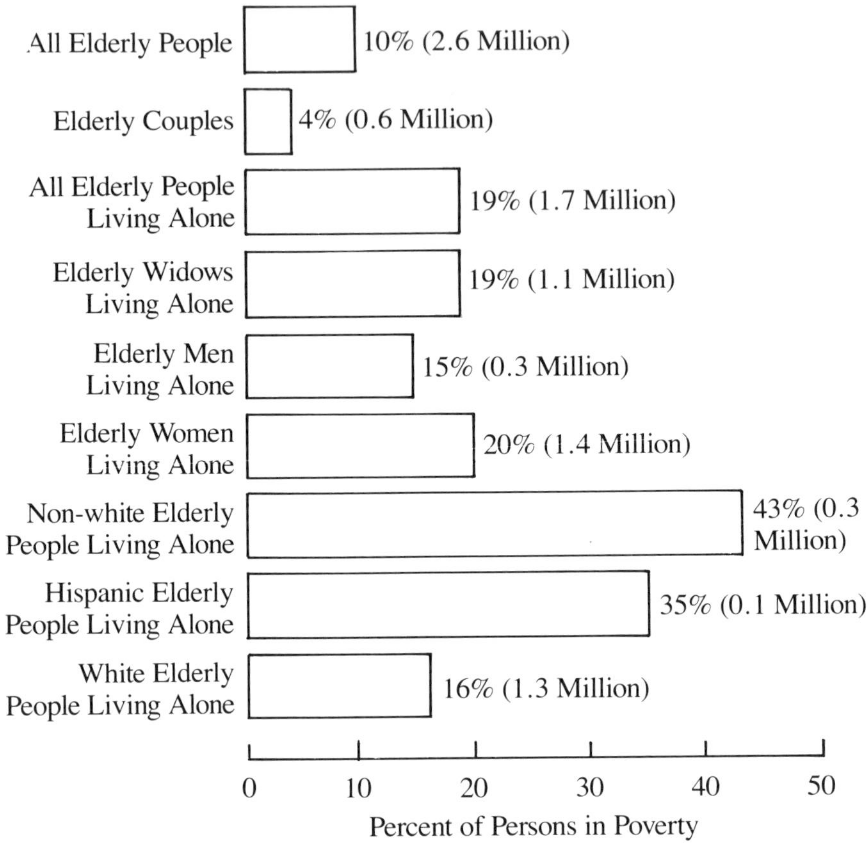

Source: ICF Estimates. "Old, Alone, and Poor: A Plan for Reducing Poverty Among Elderly People Living Alone," The Commonwealth Fund Commission on Elderly People Living Alone, Baltimore, 1987.

Special Needs of the Elderly-At-Risk

Ernestine, whose story introduced this report, exemplifies the many frail elderly whose dependency calls for personal and societal responses. These responses may involve high costs both to dependent persons and to those emotionally and geographically close to them. They also involve costs to the economy and to various community structures. Most importantly, dependency can disrupt the life plans of functionally impaired persons and their families, often impoverishing them and making it difficult for them to engage in activities to which persons generally aspire. Even the basic ADLs such as getting in and out of bed, eating and drinking, or using bathroom facilities may be overwhelming to the elderly impaired. Their caregivers in turn may find it difficult to shop, go to church, meet friends, or pursue a career.

To ameliorate the frail elderly's difficulties, even before maximizing their capabilities, individuals and society must make an investment in their lives with a range of interventions from simple affection and assistance in daily living to the provision of services associated with well-trained and competent professionals. These investments can be costly whether they involve the actual expenditure of money or the expenditure of time and energy.

At various points in the lives of the dependent elderly, these investments may be met informally within the context of families and neighborhoods, through more formal interventions, or through a combination of both. Unfortunately, not all elderly impaired persons enjoy the support of a caring, informal, social milieu. Even when this exists, it can easily be overwhelmed by the needs and demands of the disabled person. Thus, society is faced with the challenge of encouraging and supporting informal caregiving and caregivers when they are present and substituting for them when absent.

Informal Care

As noted earlier, the family provides most long term care services; unpaid relatives and friends provide 60 to 80 percent of care for impaired elderly people. Social research has dispelled the myth that families abandon their aged relatives in nursing homes.[10]

In professional jargon, family-provided long term care is usually called *informal care* or *informal supports,* in contrast to the *formal care* offered by agencies and unpaid volunteers.

Caring for an aging relative creates significant pressures on family relationships, particularly today when the family is already pressured by broad structural changes. There are more single parents, fewer children per family, and higher percentages of women in the work force. Because people are living longer, it is not unusual to see four-generation or even five-generation families. A 1982 study revealed that the average age of family members caring for frail elderly persons was 57.3 years, and that roughly a third of them are over 65.[11] Many of these persons are in poor health themselves.

Typically, the major burden of caring for the frail elderly person falls on one person in the family, usually the wife, daughter, or sister of the aging relative. When it is not a female member of the immediate family, it is likely to be a daughter-in-law, niece, or granddaughter who assumes the primary responsibility for the relative. Many women can anticipate decades of caregiving for one or another relative, even perhaps a parent or a spouse in sequence.

Strained family relationships, along with the demands of employment, are a source of pressure for women who take responsibility for an aging relative. One professional describes some of those responsible for care of an aged relative as prisoners. "You can't leave. You have someone wandering around who doesn't know where the bathroom is, who can't feed himself. No one knows what it's like unless she's been there."[12]

It is worth noting here that husbands, sons, and brothers share an equal responsibility in giving care to frail elderly family members. Even when they are not the primary direct caregivers, male relatives can offer a practical form of relief that also represents greater equity in approaching this filial duty by finding appropriate outside assistance. Both male and female relatives can establish community contacts and act as advocates with the local office on aging, home health agency, or healthcare facility, and attempt to bring together the appropriate people for the development of a logical plan of care.[13]

Even the most reliable and supportive family relationships are fragile under stress. In addition to the physical and emotional demands, some couples or families have incomes that put them in the poor or near-poor category. Family stress seems to be especially great when the older person has senile dementia. In some cases, friends and neighbors are able to help, but such assistance is not always possible and may be inadequate.

Unfortunately, the stress of caring for an elderly relative can lead to abuse of the elderly, even in their own families. Abuse of the aged is on the increase. Assaults are estimated at 1.1 million annually. Nearly six in seven (86%) of the abused aged are mistreated by their own children.[14]

The future of the family in the provision of long term care is unclear. For instance, changes in the financing and availability of long term care services and technological breakthroughs and medical advances in the treatment of intractable diseases such as Alzheimer's could have dramatic effects on the need for and demands on family caregivers. Also, as already noted, the future availability of family caregivers could be influenced by rising divorce rates, reductions in the birthrate, and increased female participation in the work force.[15]

Nevertheless, for the foreseeable future, families will remain the cornerstone of long term care.

Formal Care

Many functionally impaired elderly require a more formal set of long term care services, including adult day care, skilled home care, transportation service, and home-delivered meals. This group includes elderly persons who have no living or nearby relatives and those who depend on informal caregivers who are themselves frail, need extensive or highly technical care, or require both formal and informal support. Most of the frail elderly given substantial home care also receive some additional formal care at either personal or public expense.

In most cases, the social support system for the frail elderly comprises informal help from family and neighbors and formal services from public, private, or voluntary organizations. Whatever services are provided for the frail elderly and whatever their mode of organization, the goal should be to recognize and reinforce, not replace, the informal care and support currently provided by family and neighbors. Disruption of these informal networks of support by more extensive formal programs can work to undermine primary relationships, in addition to sometimes being more costly. At the same time, formal support systems have to be adequate to provide what families and other volunteer caregivers cannot provide, as well as to support the caregivers themselves. A proper balance needs to be maintained between the two forms of care.

Current State of Long Term Care

Unfortunately, the U.S. long term care system does not do an especially good job of maintaining this balance or of generally meeting the needs of the frail elderly. In fact, it can best be described as a "nonsystem": a set of expensive and uncoordinated programs and services that have evolved in an irregular and often patchwork manner. The sheer number of federal, state, and local programs, many of which have their own eligibility and funding arrangements, suggests the degree of complexity and confusion that exists. More than 80 programs that offer some kind of long term care assistance emanate from the federal government alone.[16]

Institutional Focus

The funding patterns of these programs are the primary determinant of what kinds of long term care services are available. For instance, the current predominance of nursing care facilities as opposed to community services in the provision of long term care services is the direct result of what Medicaid will or will not pay for. In 1984, 68 percent of Medicaid's dollars for the elderly went to nursing care facilities, 17 percent to hospitals, and 3 percent to physicians.

Medicaid finances most of the public share of nursing home costs and demands impoverishment of the elderly it helps. Home care, which is widely considered the basic service in any long term care system, derives much of its character from Medicare requirements designed for convalescence and rehabilitation following acute care. Since eligible patients must be homebound and in need of intermittent skilled services, not continuous care, Medicare's home health expenditures are focused on acute, not chronic, episodes of care. Socially oriented home care and homemaking are often provided by agencies whose staffing and procedures were developed to satisfy Medicare requirements.

Generally speaking, then, long term care services have been shaped more to respond to the requirements of government program payments than as a response to the needs of the functionally impaired elderly. The problem is made worse by the recent and almost exclusive governmental focus on cost reduction and cost control rather than on policies that first consider how best to deliver services to the frail elderly.

For instance, preliminary results of a three-year, nationwide study have found that Medicare's prospective payment system (PPS), a strategy designed to control the rate of growth in Medicare hospital payments, is forcing a shift of elderly patients from hospitals to posthospital programs. This might be acceptable if the government had prepared the programs for the additional burden. This was not done, however, and now community programs such as home health agencies, adult day care centers, hospices, and mental health centers have been overburdened, and low-income elderly unable to afford services are being squeezed out.[17]

This situation is likely to remain serious since the government has reduced Medicare hospital payments over previous estimates by more than $40 billion since 1982. As a result, the federal government has determined that more than half of the U.S. hospitals treating Medicare patients will lose money on Medicare services in 1988.[18] *Although some hospitals have closed and others are experiencing significant shortfalls, the Task Force wishes to emphasize that the sick and frail elderly, not the institutions, are potentially most at risk as a result of these payment reductions.*

The System's Effect on Ernestine

Ernestine typifies the unintended problems this "nonsystem" imposes on the elderly-at-risk. The Medicare program paid for most of Ernestine's recent hospital bill, but it still left her vulnerable to a large out-of-pocket expense that she cannot afford to pay and that possibly threatens her ability to continue to own and live in her own home. Medicare will also not pay for the many expensive medicines Ernestine requires.

Heart patients such as Ernestine are leaving hospitals earlier today, and they often need ongoing assistance at home, especially when they live alone. Medicare will not always pay for such help, however, and continuous long term care services are explicitly excluded from Medicare coverage. Medicaid might have paid the balance of Ernestine's hospital bill, but, although poor, she is ineligible for the program in her state because the value of her home exceeds Medicaid's asset allowance.

As Ernestine gets older, she will likely require additional social and supervisory help to remain in her home and avoid institutionalization. Such services, however, will not be available to her. Even if she were eligible, the Medicaid program does not pay for them. Although adamant about not leaving her home, Ernestine will almost surely have to in order to obtain the help she will require. Driven by Medicaid's eligibility requirements, she will probably have to sell her home, enter a nursing care facility, and "spend down" her remaining assets until she becomes poor enough to qualify for ongoing Medicaid assistance.

Ernestine is an elderly person who is immediately at risk because her severe personal and economic needs are not capable of being met appropriately by the present U.S. nonsystem of long term care. A proud woman who wants to remain independent may well die an institutionalized pauper.

In an ideal system of long term care, services should be client-focused and planning for them should be the combined task of the client, healthcare professionals, community agencies, and the patient's familial support group. The discontinuities in our present system of long term care, however, often do not allow this. The system is marked by many large gaps: between institutional and community-based long term care, between acute care and long term care, and between health and social services.

As a result, the elderly and their caregivers "hang on the end of the line in a kind of great social game of crack the whip: what actually happens to (them) is as likely to be the result of unintended consequences of Medicare, or Social Security, or income maintenance policy as of conscious efforts" to provide an effective set of long term care services.[19]

Long Term Care Personnel

An analysis of the current state of long term care must include a discussion of the cadre of caregivers that it employs. Inevitably, the quantity, makeup, and quality of long term care personnel influence the care and lives of the frail elderly for better or worse.

The predominantly female paraprofessionals who provide primary healthcare and housekeeping services for people both in their homes and in institutions perform what relatives of the frail elderly would consider humanly valuable work, but these jobs are neither highly paid nor highly respected. Many who provide these crucial services in our cities are black and Hispanic women who are the primary wage earners in their own families. Likewise, aides in nursing care facilities and personal care facilities, again primarily women, do physically and emotionally demanding work for disproportionately low wages. These persons are often in positions of enormous responsibility.Greater investment needs to be made in their orientation, ongoing training, and wages.

The critical shortage of registered nurses (RNs) is well known. The problem of recruitment is compounded in long term care, where nursing positions command lower salaries and are perceived as having less status than positions in acute care settings. A recent survey of staffing needs by the American Health Care Association found that 58 percent of responding nursing homes had RN vacancies and that 50 percent said it would take at least 3 months to fill those vacancies.[20] In relation to the projected need in long term care, shortages are anticipated in occupational and physical therapy staff as well.

Further, geriatric nursing educators are concerned about the gap between projected needs for master's level geriatric nurse-specialists and the small numbers that are currently in preparation. Even if a redistribution of nurses from hospitals to nursing homes was realistic, the numbers of properly prepared professionals would not be available, nor would the salaries attract them.

Although an increasingly high percentage of the patients that physicians care for are 65 and older, very few physicians are trained in geriatrics. The multiple, chronic illnesses that elderly persons develop and the relationship of these conditions to their social and economic situation call for a different style of practicing medicine than most specialists are accustomed to performing. The dominant style of medical care is marked by short term intervention with the expectation that the patient's condition will improve. Many elderly patients, however, have a complex of gradually debilitating conditions without the residue of health and strength to "get better." Traditional medical specialties do not dispose a physician to address this complex problem of interrelated illnesses. Geriatric specialists are in a position to offer leadership in elderly care. The body of knowledge and practical experience in chronic care developed in long term care settings can also be called upon to enhance care of the frail elderly in hospital settings.

Toward More Humane and Effective Long Term Care

This chapter's description of the frail elderly's special requirements, i.e., their need for a variety of coordinated informal and formal supports tailored to their preferences and to the degree and extent of their functional impairment, underscores the fact that existing long term care policies are exacting a heavy toll on today's frail elderly and are wholly inadequate for the task of meeting the nation's expanding future responsibilities in this area. This situation forces the question, "How can we create policies to provide more humane and effective long term care?"

The answer to that question is especially difficult since long term care means different things to different people. It is generally misunderstood, even by some healthcare professionals. For instance, the general public too easily equates all long term care with nursing care facilities. On the other hand, in dealing with elderly patients who are not sick enough to remain in the hospital but are too ill to live by themselves, some hospital staffs believe long term care means a temporary or permanent nursing home placement or a support service provided at home. For federal or state policymakers, long term care might conjure up the uncomfortable specter of runaway costs in existing or proposed programs. For still others, long term care for the frail elderly may mean the exploitation of a new market to enhance personal and corporate wealth.

To an important degree this definitional confusion is itself a reflection of the present system's discontinuities; its financing mechanisms, strong institutional biases, and fragmented character exercise a powerful hegemony over our thinking by inclining us to construe long term care services as a series of single, disconnected events of hospitalization, nursing facility care, home care, or other discrete interventions.

A New Definition of Long Term Care

The Task Force believes that a more humane definition of long term care begins with the needs and preferences of the functionally impaired elderly person. Viewed from this client-oriented perspective, long term care is understood as an extended transition from one functional state to another. Its primary objective is to ensure that the frail elderly person receives the mix of formal and informal services appropriate to his or her needs.

This definition recognizes that *all* care of the elderly is long term care and that services are not distinct and separate but interchangeable. For instance, some frail elderly can be served at home, others in a congregate housing complex with additional in-house services, and still others in a nursing care facility. Moreover, community services such as transportation, day care, delivered meals, and home care can be combined in various ways. Even institutions such as hospitals and nursing care facilities can theoretically mix the services they provide with other services available in the community.[21]

Thus, long term care is a hybrid—part health and part social services. It refers not to the places where services are offered, or to the programs that provide them, or to "market opportunities," but rather to the array of services that are required to compensate an elderly individual for functional problems. This client-oriented focus recognizes that the frail elderly, like other citizens, are human beings who have an ongoing need for a variety of social goods such as adequate income, housing, healthcare, and recreational opportunities. It also recognizes the special needs of their caregivers.

But the mere existence and availability of an array of services are not by themselves a sufficient guarantee that the needs of the frail elderly will be met in a timely or appropriate manner. The current long term care system provides a range of valuable and expensive services: Social Security and Supplemental Security Income (SSI) provide income support; Medicare makes acute and postacute care available; the Older Americans Act supports a variety of community services; and Medicaid provides nursing home care. Since each of these programs is distinct, however, in that each has a different set of eligibility and funding arrangements, a serious fragmentation in service delivery too often results.

Ernestine's case drives this point home. She is known to a number of health and social service providers. But none of the providers is capable of taking responsibility for organizing and monitoring a program of care for her. Each provider's focus is too narrow to consider the full range of Ernestine's functional and environmental needs over time. The current system's discontinuities are likely to cause her to enter a nursing care facility and therefore be cut off from timely and appropriate access to other health and social services.

Ernestine's example could be multiplied repeatedly. Her situation and the innumerable others like hers highlight the critical importance of developing *integrating elements* within each community and health care institution. These will allow a client-centered program of long term care to mix and match available services to support the frail elderly as they move from one functional state to another.

Long Term Care as a Continuum of Care

The Task Force believes that the infusion into long term care of an explicit client focus, the availability of an array of effective long term care services, and the provision of certain integrating elements can best be envisioned as a coordinated *continuum of care*. A successful continuum of care has three essential features:

- *Client Focus:* It is "user friendly"; i.e., its primary focus is on the needs and preferences of those being served. Clients are the reason for its being. Elderly individuals and caregivers, as a group, are slower to ask for help such as healthcare. But once they do, their need is urgent and they find that continued navigation of the current system of long term care is a difficult venture at best. A true continuum of care is actively responsible for anticipating and assessing the frail elderly's needs and seeing them through each site and level of care and support over time.
- *Services:* The continuum is more than a collection of services located in the same community or related to the same organization. The range of services is comprehensive and covers the spectrum from social intensive, community based, primarily outpatient care to health intensive, institution based, primarily inpatient care. In a continuum, each type of care provider has a significant role in providing services for the elderly. No institution or agency has a greater role; all are required if the needs of the elderly are to be met appropriately and in the most suitable and cost-effective environment. By providing continuity of care, the continuum focuses on prevention and early intervention for those who have been identified as high risk and provides easy transition from service to service as needs change.

- *Integrating Elements:* To operate these services on a day-to-day basis as a continuum of care, the additional step of providing key integrating elements is *essential*. The integrating elements ensure that the continuum remains focused on the client and avoids competing and conflicting programs, communication gaps, budget conflicts, autonomously functioning programs, and multiproduct marketing. The integrating elements (described next) also help to maximize the efficient use of scarce resources, both human and financial.

It is the integrating elements providing the coordination between and among services which distinguish a true continuum from other sets of services simply having an information and referral system. Without the coordination, there is no continuum. Finally, the integrating elements require each service provider to network or collaborate with many other community and/or healthcare agencies that are different from its own.

The following integrating elements comprise the bridge between clients and services:

- *Planning:* A commitment to coordinated community-wide planning is required for any successful continuum of care. The governing boards and top management of each service in the continuum and appropriate medical staffs should be involved in the development of the continuum of care's strategic plan. Managers and staff at all levels also need to be involved as appropriate.
- *Care Management:* Another key integrating element is a care management program. The term "care management" is sometimes referred to as "case management" or "managed care." The Task Force believes there is a significant difference. "Managed care" or "case management" has recently been converted by government and other third-party payors from a method of managing patient care into a method of controlling the cost of care in acute settings. *Care* management, on the other hand, refers to a process for assessing both the short and the long term healthcare and social services needed to meet the needs of a functionally impaired person. *Case* management is cost-centered and episodic; *care* management is person-centered and long term. Care management involves development of a support system that selects, on an as-needed basis, from an array of services within the continuum. It consists of several basic components: screening, functional assessment, family and caregiver needs assessment, care planning and team conferencing, program eligibility determination, service referral and procurement, monitoring and tracking, and reassessment.
- *Management Information System:* A management information system (usually a computerized communication system) should

access and integrate data from all the services in the continuum. The result increases both accuracy in historical data and scrutiny of functional levels and integrates health and social service data with financial data.

- *Financing:* In order for continuum budgeting to be effective and efficient, all providers must participate in the budgeting process. This facilitates planning and enables revenues from strong programs to be used to supplement necessary but financially weaker ones such as the care management function. Pooling program funds will also make savings possible due to economies of scale and operational efficiencies. In this regard, capitated financing theoretically offers incentives to develop a continuum: flexibility in choosing the most appropriate service, minimal billing/collection efforts, and means to limit total expenditures for healthcare.
- *Administrative Structure:* The organizational leadership is the single element that connects all the others in achieving a successful continuum. The leadership enables the people within separate services to perceive themselves as belonging to one integrated organization and is able to convey a clear vision of the continuum. Through joint planning, identification of problems, and sharing of information, the administrative structure is able to coordinate the numerous services and support systems within the continuum. The communication channels should flow in all directions: the boards of directors, staffs, physicians, and community must understand the direction and progress of the continuum through task forces, committees, management meetings, newsletters, etc.

Community-Wide Collaboration

In summary, the success or failure of a continuum depends on the willingness of providers, volunteer and community organizations, and administrators to collaborate and create a truly *integrated* network. The frail elderly are thus enabled to move within the continuum as their functional and environmental needs change, and the continuum responds quickly to these changes.

Ideally, the continuum offers a mix of basic, supportive, and remedial services to compensate the frail elderly for functional impairments in the areas of social, economic, mental, physical, and self-care activity.

The Task Force is not offering a prescriptive formula for creating a continuum of care, but rather is setting forth the elements that any successful continuum should contain. Since each community's long term care needs are different, each continuum will be unique and illustrative of that particular community's makeup and needs.

One way of graphically depicting the continuum of care is shown in Figure 2. There may be other and better ways to portray the continuum, but the Task Force believes that this figure emphasizes the dynamic relationships that should exist between an array of formal and informal services, as well as the necessary integrating elements in a client-centered continuum of care.

FIGURE 2

Example of a Continuum for Long Term Care

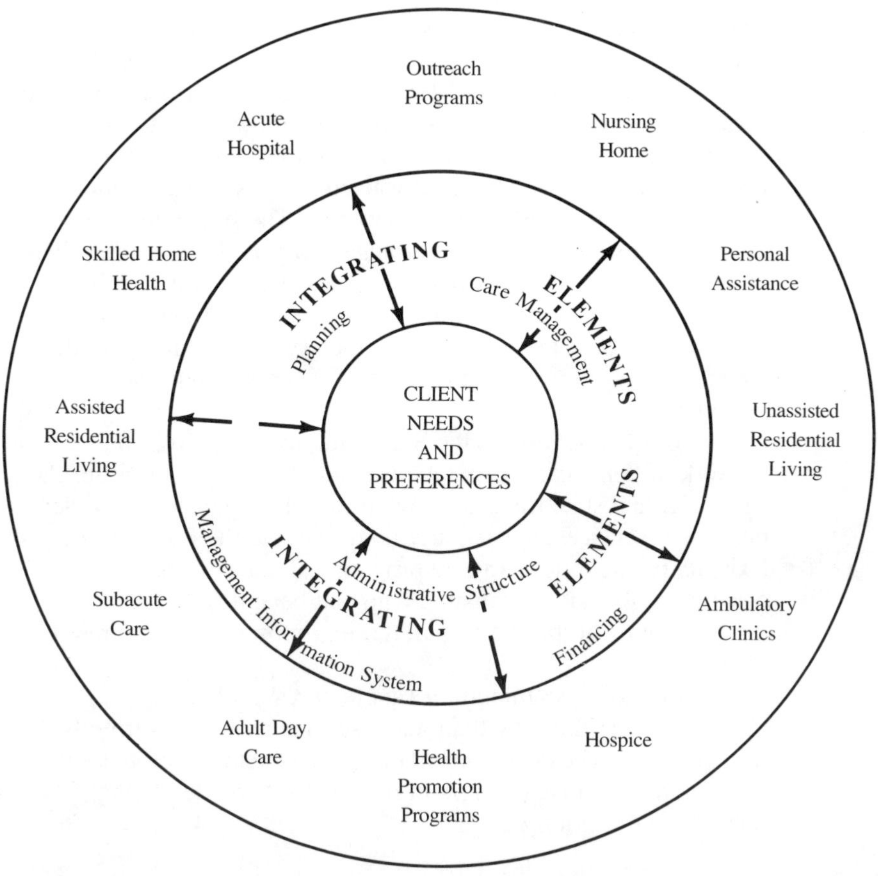

Obstacles to a Continuum of Care

As desirable as a comprehensive and integrated system of long term care service is, several significant barriers stand in the way of its adoption. Among the most important is a widespread and misguided prejudice that fails to acknowledge that resource expenditure on behalf of the frail elderly can be productive. Research and experience have demonstrated that many infirmities of old age are *not* inevitable and can be reversed. The failure to recognize these facts is a form of ageism that has ramifications for program planning and can inhibit professionals in a variety of disciplines from specializing in care of the elderly.

Community leaders and healthcare professionals who are grappling with how to organize and provide services to their frail elderly in the context of a continuum of care face several other obstacles:

- Medicare and Medicaid funding and eligibility arrangements artificially separate acute and long term care, preventing flexibility in the delivery of services. However, some states recently have made efforts to overcome this obstacle by creatively using Medicaid waivers to narrow the chasm that currently exists. Section 2176 of the 1981 Omnibus Budget Reconciliation Act permitted the Department of Health and Human Services to waive certain Medicaid requirements in order to allow states to finance a broad range of community-based long term care services. In Oregon, for instance, Medicaid-waivered funds and state funds are used to purchase home care and day care. The state purchases home care directly and makes arrangements partly to finance live-in care. The case manager does the assessment and determines the amount of services and, therefore, the amount of money that the program will pay; these monies are then provided directly to the client to defray a portion of the cost of an approved privately hired provider.

  In Massachusetts, the State Unit on Aging created a network of home care corporations using the Older Americans Act, Title XX, and state funds to provide case management and other purchased services, particularly home care, to the frail elderly.
- Existing public long term care programs all have strong constituencies that are satisfied with and benefit from the discontinuities of the status quo; these groups are likely to resist change.
- The concept of a continuum of care requires a different management philosophy than many service providers currently have in place. The development of a new system therefore requires major administrative changes in planning for and delivering services to the elderly.

- There is a general lack of experience and knowledge among healthcare professionals about the development and management of a continuum of care. Most formal programs of healthcare administration have only recently introduced long term and ambulatory care as elective programs. Few professional development programs have been available in this area for current administrative personnel.
- Continuum of care requires healthcare providers to plan and work with other service providers in the community. Traditionally, many healthcare facilities have been able to plan programs and services in isolation from other groups. An effective continuum of care must be developed in partnership with other providers and/or community agencies. The continuum also requires a team approach to care that can identify and address a wider range of problems than might be uncovered by a single practitioner. Healthcare providers espouse the team concept for care in their current environments; the continuum of care requires that it be expanded to the community when planning and delivering services to meet the increasing needs of the elderly-at-risk.

The continuum of care, with its explicit client focus, array of services, and integrating elements, is a powerful concept that frees our thinking about care of the elderly from its moorings in the narrower confines of existing policies and programs. By adding clarity and shape to our thinking about better ways of addressing the frail elderly's functional needs, the continuum of care enables us to critique current governmental and private sector long term care arrangements, understand how these too often excessively, if unintentionally, burden the elderly and their caregivers, and appreciate the urgent need for fundamental reform.

In Chapters 3 and 4 of this report, the Task Force will examine how the various ministries of the Church, parishes, dioceses, Catholic Charities agencies, healthcare facilities, and state Catholic conferences have an important and vital role to play in improving service delivery to the frail elderly and their caregivers. The Task Force will make recommendations in the areas of Church and community leadership; additions to and improvements in the provision of pastoral, health, and social services; and advocacy at the state and federal levels.

In Chapter 5, the Task Force examines the critical role that government, especially the federal government, must play in creating policies to provide more humane and effective long term care.

Moral Vision

The CHA Task Force believes that fundamental long term care reform will remain an elusive goal unless it is firmly anchored in a set of values about the frail elderly and their functional needs. Societal agreement on such a set of values constitutes a shared moral vision that can become the basis for and the animating force behind needed changes in our long term care system. Creative programs of reform are the result of bringing a constructive moral vision to bear on a clear understanding of the problem.

The next chapter locates the basic elements of that moral vision in Scripture, Church tradition, Catholic social thought, and in our common experience of human need.

Catholic social principles have evolved over the last 100 years in response to the various forms of human pain and alienation occasioned by the development of modern industrial society. They derive most basically from the belief that human dignity is rooted in each person's relationship with a transcendent God; its clearest and most tangible expression is in caring human communities, especially those that reflect solidarity with society's most vulnerable members.[22]

Thus, Catholic social thought recognizes that all of the Church's work in pursuit of justice is designed to foster the social and economic conditions that promote the dignity of human beings. As this chapter has indicated, our fragmented system of long term care has effectively pushed many of the elderly to the edges of modern society. The frail elderly who live alone and are poor are especially vulnerable. A society that neglects its weakest citizens is itself in need of social, economic, and moral realignment.

This moral vision necessarily speaks most powerfully to the Catholic community. It is not limited to a Catholic audience alone, however, since the values on which it relies are reflected in our nation's broader Judeo-Christian and humanistic tradition. This tradition also aspires to recognize all human beings, including the frail elderly, as brothers and sisters and to recognize its obligation to assist them.

The next chapter will draw on the major themes of Catholic social teaching to identify our responsibilities to the frail elderly, especially those who are poor, and to help each of us shape more effective personal, social, and institutional responses to their basic human needs.

NOTES

1. The trends reported here are based on data from the U.S. Census Bureau in 1983.
2. Jack M. Guralnik, Dwight B. Brock, and Jacob A. Brody, "The Changing Demography of the Elderly in the United States," unpublished research paper, Bethesda, MD, National Institute on Aging, 1986.
3. Guralnik et al.
4. J. Strong, *Caring for America's Alzheimer's Victims,* Hearings before the Select Committee on Aging, May 21, 1985, House of Representatives, 99th Congress, Washington, DC, U.S. Government Printing Office, 1985.
5. D. Mechanic, "Challenges in Long Term Care Policy," *Health Affairs,* Summer 1987, p. 23.
6. Rosalie A. Kane and Robert L. Kane, *Long Term Care: Principles, Programs, and Policies,* New York, Springer Publishing Co., 1987, p. 24.

7. Anne Somers, "Insurance for Long Term Care: Some Definitions, Problems, and Guidelines for Action," *New England Journal of Medicine,* Vol. 317, no. 1, July 2, 1987.
8. "Old, Alone and Poor: A Plan for Reducing Poverty Among Elderly People Living Alone," The Commonwealth Fund Commission on Elderly People Living Alone, Baltimore, 1987.
9. Robyn Stone, *The Feminization of Poverty and Older Women: An Update,* Washington, DC, U.S. Department of Health and Human Services, February 1986.
10. Gail Lee Cafferata, Judith Sangl, and Robyn Stone, *Caregivers of the Frail Elderly: A National Profile,* The National Center for Health Services Research, 1982.
11. Cafferata et al., pp. 4, 11.
12. Clare Ansberry, "Family Affair: Abuse of the Elderly by Their Own Children Increases in America," *Wall Street Journal,* Feb. 3, 1988, p. 1.
13. See Philip W. Brickner et al., *Long Term Health Care: Providing A Spectrum of Services To The Aged,* New York, Basic Books, 1987, pp. 199 onward.
14. Ansberry.
15. Brickner et al.
16. Kane and Kane, p. 71.
17. *American Medical News,* Jan. 15, 1988, p. 29.
18. *Medicare Prospective Payment and the American Health Care System: Report to the Congress, June 1988,* Washington, DC, Prospective Payment Assessment Commission, p. 5.
19. Marion Ein Lewin, ed., *Health Policy Agenda: Some Critical Questions,* Washington, DC, American Enterprise Institute Studies in Health Policies, 1985, pp. 115-116.
20. Van Ellet, "The Nursing Home Shortage: Which Providers Are Suffering Most?" *Provider,* March 1988, pp. 34-35.
21. This definition is derived in part from material developed by Kane and Kane.
22. See David J. O'Brien and Thomas A. Shannon, *Renewing the Earth,* Catholic Documents on Peace, Justice and Liberation, New York, Image/Doubleday, 1977; and *Economic Justice for All,* Pastoral Letter on Catholic Social Teaching and the U.S. Economy, Washington, DC, National Conference of Catholic Bishops, 1986.

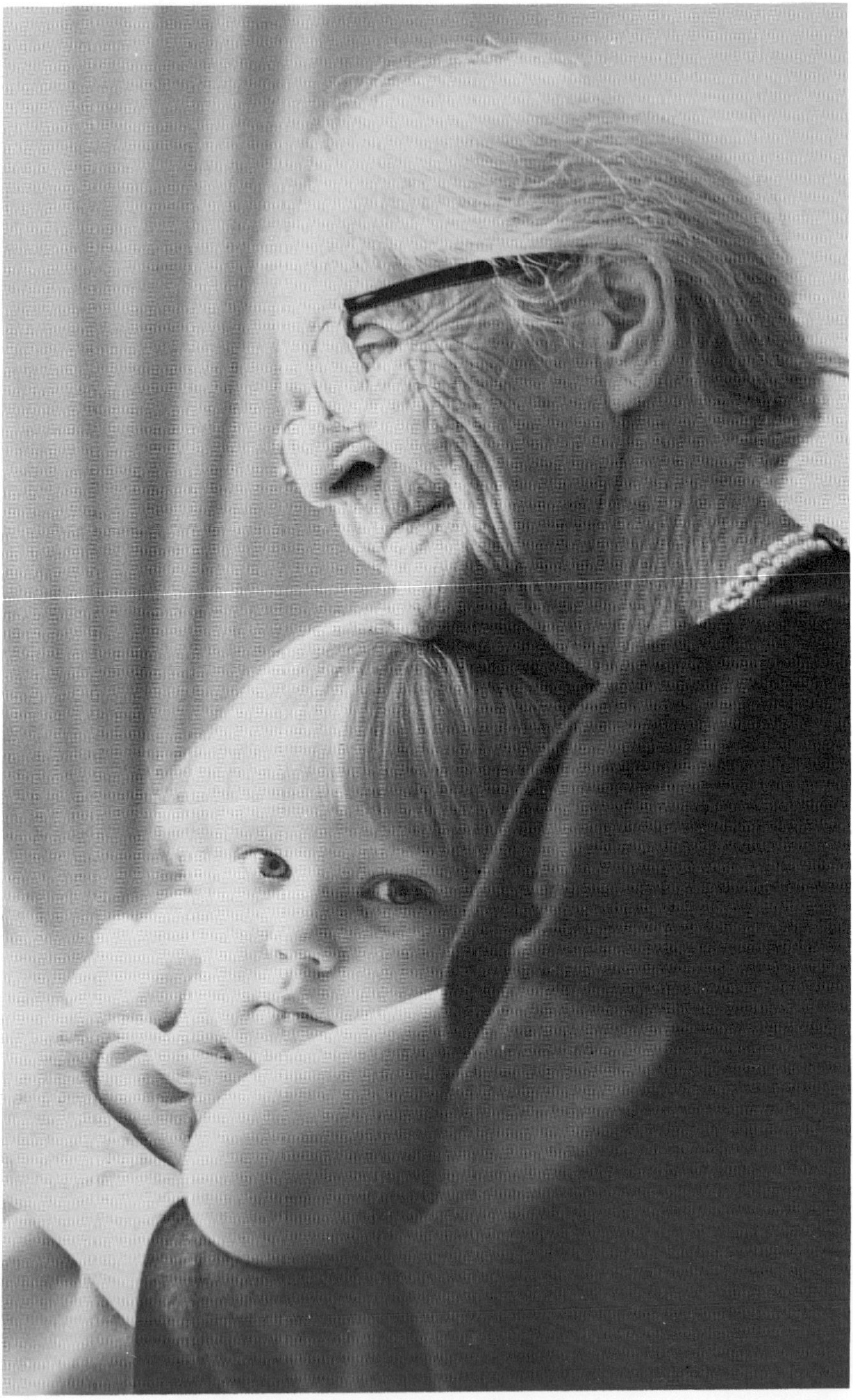

2

A Reflection in Faith

The Theological Background of the Church's Concern for the Elderly

Introduction: A Sacrament of God's Presence

Any theological reflection by the Catholic healthcare ministry on its responsibility to the elderly-at-risk begins with the call of Jesus Christ to share his healing mission—a call issued within the human community through the lives of the elderly themselves, particularly those who are most vulnerable. The familiar Gospel theme of a shared journey suggests that the elderly themselves have much to share with the community and that younger members ought to include them in their lives and support them when their health fails.

Sharing the human journey also suggests that healthcare providers should work within their facilities and with others in the community to build coordinated, accessible, and client-focused programs of care for the frail elderly. These programs should provide what the elderly need and at the same time allow them and their caregivers the freedom to decide for themselves what services they need to take advantage of. Finally, this theological image of a shared journey suggests that there has to be a public policy framework in the United States based on a commitment to the common good of all citizens. Basic principles of Catholic social teaching help to translate this ideal into more explicit social and economic commitments to the well-being of the elderly and indeed to each of us.

God Cries Out to Us in the Midst of Life

In the midst of a frantic and self-seeking culture, one can find consolation in the fact that in all situations, whether they be filled with anxiety or peace, despair or hope, life cries out to people. There is an urging, a call that Catholics and other people of faith identify as the call of God. Whoever hears it and responds is empowered to make visible the invisible love of God. Thus, the care and concern that people exhibit for one another and their communities is not theirs alone. It is a sharing in divine care.

Christians believe further that the life of Jesus revealed God's care among people. Christ heard the cry of the hungry and and broke bread with them. He heard the cry of the rich and called them to generosity. He heard the cry of the sick and reached out to the paralyzed man (Mk 2:5), put his hand on the fevered head of Peter's mother-in-law (Mk 1:31), and grappled with the boy writhing on the ground (Mk 2:97). Through all these compassionate gestures of Jesus, we believe that the love of God entered human life. That is why Jesus was called the "image of the invisible God" (Col 1:15). Some are bold enough to think that when human beings do the same, the ministry of Jesus is continued and the love of the invisible, intangible God can be seen and touched in this world.

The human voice of God can be heard today in a special way, calling each person to make His love and compassion visible in the lives of the elderly, many of whom face the prospect of poor health, poverty, and abandonment. In this regard, the responsibility of persons who value them is threefold. First, whatever can be done must be done to make it possible for the elderly-at-risk to remain self-sufficient and participating members of their communities. Second, as they become frail and increasingly dependent, positive attitudes toward frailty that spring from our Catholic values need to be shared and reinforced. Additional supports need to be made available that will enable them to choose the living arrangement most appropriate for them. Given more defined and consistent help, most frail elderly persons can remain relatively self-sufficient. For those who do require institutional care, it is important to enable them to experience the sense of personal dignity that comes with the retention of some measure of control and decision-making responsibility in their lives. Finally, our faith tradition urges us to help the elderly find new ways in which they can contribute to the spiritual growth of their families and communities.

Human Life Is a Journey Shared

The perennial image of the pilgrimage is a powerful model of the Christian life. It suggests appropriate ways of responding to God's call to live in ways that include, rather than exclude, the elderly. A pilgrimage is a journey that individuals make alone and yet together. It is a journey to a holy place, accompanied by a holy presence. Throughout a pilgrimage, the pilgrims are called forth by people and events to grow, to learn to care, to stretch in service of each other and of God. In other words, a pilgrimage is a call to continual conversion.

The elderly are very often themselves signs of continual conversion in the midst of the community. By remaining open to new challenges, many of them have found their later years to be enriching and creative in new, valuable ways. Some have taken on child-caring responsibilities. Many have provided other kinds of support to their families and friends. Many have found opportunities to share with their parishes or communities their years of experience and professional competence.

Many, even after they have lost their capacity for certain kinds of physical activity, have continued to develop their intellectual and spiritual gifts and to share these with others. All major religious traditions are filled with reminders that elderly persons are the present generation's link to the past. Through the experiences they share, the elderly play an indispensable role as mediators of the traditions of faith, endurance, and human achievement that help to sustain their children in the present and inspire hope in their grandchildren. By persevering in the struggle to accept the losses that many elderly people suffer—economic security, status, relationships, health—they can offer a unique witness to human dignity and the inner life of the spirit.

The Inner Journey

The spiritual pilgrimage followed by each elderly person is, of course, unique. Certain characteristic features, however, arise from common life circumstances. Most experience the major vocational changes of retirement from a career and diminishment of their family-raising responsibilities. Because of these and other changes, it is typical for the elderly to have more leisure time. On the other hand, they typically suffer the loss of social and economic status attached to these productive roles. They also often suffer declining health, particularly as they grow older.

Lived circumstances are bound to shape spirituality as we age. With more leisure we have the responsibility to reflect, to deepen our prayer life, and to give ourselves in service. Age often brings with it the difficult call to learn how to find redemption in chronic pain, loneliness, and the prospect of death. Other community members need to be sensitive to the burdens of the elderly and their potential contribution to the spiritual richness of the community.

An Invitation to Community

The call of God invites individuals to become a people, a community in which all belong to and care for each other. This vision of life values human solidarity and the participation of all, including the poor and the frail, in community life. It also implies a commitment to building family and community relationships. This vision clashes with the many forms of individualism that so often lead to conflict and social disintegration in modern society. It also challenges forms of isolation that prevent the elderly from participating in a common social and cultural world with younger, more self-sufficient members of society. When persons are isolated, whether in neighborhoods, parishes, or institutions, the human bonds that can only be forged in the sharing of ordinary life experiences are threatened.

The Call to Intergenerational Solidarity

On the other hand, when people are faithful to God's call, when they remain true to their pilgrim existence, they build communities of families and individuals in solidarity with each other. This enables the members to offer daily expressions of faith and hope to each other. They enrich each other in wisdom and in compassion simply by being present with one another. Together, then, people can come to accept aging as a gift as well as a challenge that enhances the quality of each person's life, even in those instances when they must share with each other the burden that diminishment of physical or mental powers inevitably brings.

This call to intergenerational solidarity and the moral commitments implicit in it urge responsible persons to work together to heal institutional and social dislocations that add to the burdens of growing old in our society today. Some of that effort will take place within families and communities in very personal ways. An important part of it also has to be done organizationally, often through institutions. A commitment to intergenerational solidarity should also find expression in public policy regarding the elderly.

Finding God and Each Other in Frailty

The elderly who suffer significant physical and sometimes mental impairment are at the heart of the Church's concern because they are often the most isolated and the most vulnerable to exploitation and neglect. Those who embrace them in their vulnerability show a willingness to be led toward their own conversion.

Their often feeble bodies summon younger persons back to fundamental human and religious truths. Among these is the belief that a way exists to find in the heart of the loneliness and dependence that come with aging, a deepening of family relationships, and new levels of intimacy with God. Pope John Paul II urges that "our desire must be that the prayers of the elderly fill the home, and their extraordinary capacity for evangelization be an impulse for the vigor of love and affection, an orientation for the fundamental values of existence."[1]

An encounter with a frail person has the potential to provide younger persons with the courage to face their own future debilitation, loss of independence, and death, and to find redemption in these experiences. By their presence, frail elderly invite others to yield a measure of independence. In doing so, they offer them a relationship that actualizes the call to become one with each other and with God, who unites all believers. By sharing their journey of faith, younger, more self-sufficient persons can learn something about the kind of security and peace that is gained only through fully entrusting oneself to the One who loves each person unconditionally.

Christians Are Called to Relieve Pain and Isolation

The most loving and compassionate families will be increasingly sensitive to their aging relatives who experience gradual debilitation and daily physical pain and anxiety. As it becomes more difficult for aging persons to manage routine tasks, their living space becomes smaller. It shrinks even further when they find themselves constantly fighting their preoccupation with incapacity and physical pain.

Younger, healthier persons sometimes shun the frail elderly, finding it uncomfortable to listen to the voice of pain and loneliness. Many old persons, however, fear abandonment and social isolation more than anything. Their fear of losing their minds, of being institutionalized, and of dying is primarily a fear of losing contact with those they love. Yet within a perspective of faith, no one is ever alone. The fundamental dignity of each human being derives from God's faithful relationship with him or her. The members of a community of faith can witness to these persons' dignity and to God's fidelity by staying with them as their health and strength fail.

Many elderly live for years with chronic diseases and with great pain. All life speaks of God's love, but the voice of God often speaks loudest in the midst of pain. When people of faith share with those in pain, they are sometimes privileged to hear God's voice. They are slowly able to help those in pain to hear what God may be saying. When others share with them their faith, they share the conviction that no one suffers alone. All suffer in union with the One who died for all and who gives meaning and grace to their pain. The sacramental life of the Church is particularly important to those in pain. The Anointing of the Sick makes the redemptive value of our care explicit and joins the suffering person to the healing presence of Jesus Christ. The Eucharist reunites us in the community celebration of the death and resurrection of Jesus, literally providing food for the journey.

Christian Acceptance of Death

Christians see death as something more than the end of life; it is also a way to the fullness of life. They believe that their pilgrimage with others in this life leads more deeply into the life of God and that people learn throughout life how to yield gracefully to God at the time of death. In death, the relationships with people they have loved are broken, only to be transformed. People of faith yield themselves in complete trust, in the most intimate of all relationships, to God. Death is for Christians apparently the end, but simultaneously the moment when the present is transformed into the fullness of life.

Catholic Social Teaching: Institutions and Social Policy

If the Church's special concern for the elderly-at-risk is to be practical and effective, its efforts must go beyond family, parish, and neighborhood commitments. The Church and those who carry out institutional ministries in its name have to develop more effective and better integrated health and social programs. Practical concern also requires that Catholic leaders be advocates in public forums for adequate government protection and support of these vulnerable citizens.

Catholic social teaching has been clear about the need for social action when the well-being of people is at risk. "(T)he teachings of the Church insist the *government has a moral function: protecting human rights and securing basic justice for all members of the commonwealth* . . . More specifically, it is the responsibility of all citizens, acting through their government, to assist and empower the poor, the disadvantaged, the handicapped, and the unemployed."[2]

Basic justice in this context encompasses commutative justice, which calls for fundamental fairness in social and economic transactions; distributive justice, which demands the allocation of resources in such a way as to ensure that the necessary economic needs of all are met; and social or contributive justice, which requires that all contribute to the well-being of society and that social and economic structures foster the active participation of everyone.

One of the central themes of Catholic social teaching is that human dignity is manifest in our ability to reason and understand, in our freedom to shape our own lives and the life of our communities, and in our capacity for love and friendship.[3] Each of us has a responsibility to help the elderly give concrete expression to their personal dignity by developing and offering them ways to exercise freedom of choice and to participate meaningfully in the life of the community insofar as they are able.

Within institutional settings and service delivery systems, healthcare and social service professionals can promote the dignity of clients by establishing a specific client focus and an integrated set of services and by eliminating rigid barriers to the exercise of the clients' self-determination. Many of these impediments are designed primarily for reasons of organizational efficiency and convenience. The only legitimate constraints on the autonomy of clients are those that are the inevitable result of physical and mental disability and those which are dictated by the physical safety of the person, the rights of others, and the need for order in communal living situations. Within these bounds, the elderly person should be allowed as much opportunity for choice as possible.

Government also has a role in protecting those political and economic rights that are required by individual dignity. Among the basic economic rights that undergird human dignity are the right to food, clothing, shelter, and medical care.[4] Government should create systems of accountability through law and regulation that protect the rights of individuals without creating onerous financial and bureaucratic systems that can undermine the very patterns of care fostering human dignity.

One of the other primary responsibilities of government at all levels is to promote the common good, a formidable task in a pluralistic—even individualistic—society. Recent Catholic social teaching has insisted that because healthcare is so fundamental to human well-being, healthcare is one of those basic goods that government has a responsibility to ensure all its citizens. The Church's position is that need ought to be the measure of individual access and overall allocation of available resources.

If basic need is understood as the determining criterion for access and allocation, then what has come to be known in the Church as the "preferential option for the poor" becomes a means to establishing more equitable patterns of participation in the healthcare system. At present, some people have few if *any* options regarding healthcare for themselves or their families. The "preferential option" would demand the inclusion of those who are at present excluded, even at some cost to others. It would no longer be morally legitimate to limit the cost of healthcare for some groups and payers by limiting the access of other groups. When the Church speaks for the poor and assesses institutional practice and public policy from the perspective of its effect on their lives, it is only urging a more adequate expression of the common good.

The same concern on the part of the Church for the dignity of the individual and the common good urges active promotion of the just treatment of workers, a central theme of the social encyclicals from the beginning. Just treatment of healthcare workers implies a recognition of their right to adequate training, to a just wage, and to the formation of associations to advance their legitimate interests in the workplace.[5]

The principle of *subsidiarity,* also drawn from the Church's social teaching, should be useful in conceptualizing appropriate relationships among individuals, agencies, and government bodies in the provision of services for the elderly. Subsidiarity requires that formal delivery systems and government intervention not attempt to supplant what individuals, families, and local groups can accomplish by their own enterprise and industry. It also "guarantees institutional pluralism. It provides space for freedom, initiative, and creativity on the part of many social agents. At the same time it insists that *all* these agents should work in ways to build up the social body."[6]

Individuals should be encouraged in the interests of subsidiarity to maintain healthy lifestyles and to provide financially for their future care needs. Families also should assume some responsibility for the care of their aging relatives and participate in planning ways to cover the costs of formal care in the eventuality that it becomes necessary. Formal systems of care should be designed to help individuals and families carry the burden of disability and to provide what they are not able to provide themselves. These systems should be made up of a variety of agencies working in concert with each other to provide what is in the best interest of the elderly in the communities they serve. Government policy and programming should favor initiatives that are designed to support informal caregiving, while protecting from abandonment persons who are without family and financial resources.

Conclusion

Our movement through life is a continual call to conversion, a call to compassionate caring for each other. It is a call to community. Since everyone is moving toward a shared life together, no one should ever be abandoned. The elderly who, for reasons of frailty and economic vulnerability, are at risk can lead us in life's journey. Disregard for their plight is a denial of the deepest meaning of life as we understand it.

The Church should be present at all levels of intervention on behalf of the elderly, especially those who are frail, alone, and poor. Otherwise, our exhortations to accompany one another, to be just in our relationships, to treat all with dignity, to reach out in compassion, only add to the burden of the elderly by raising false expectations and leading to unfulfilled hopes. For us, too, hopes will remain unfulfilled, for we shall have missed the call of God among us.

Long Term Care: Values and Goals

The preceding articulation of the theological basis for the Church's interest in and concern about aging led the Task Force to be guided by the following set of values and goals:

- Respect for human dignity requires that any program or system of long term care nurture the autonomy of elderly clients by building in as much opportunity for personal choice as is possible. Respect for the functionally impaired demands that their choices and social opportunities not be artificially limited.

- A sense of personal responsibility should urge each person to take reasonable care of his or her health and to take steps to contribute financially to the cost of possible future dependency.
- The elderly, particularly once they become frail, should be ensured access to an adequate range and mix of services, which should be individually available to them on the basis of need, not economic status. In the interests of making the system practically accessible, there has to be clear communication and coordination among the organizations that finance, regulate, and provide the services.
- Long term care programs and policies should recognize the central role played by families in the provision of care and should support and supplement what families are able to provide rather than attempt to substitute for it. Community caregiving and volunteerism should be encouraged.
- Financing arrangements should be designed to support informal caregivers' efforts and to cover those persons whose families are not able to assume responsibility for them and those who have no family.
- Adequate professional preparation and equitable incomes should be ensured for long term care personnel.
- Policy should foster public accountability for the accessibility, quality, and cost of all services, whether offered under private or public auspices.

This set of values and goals forms the basis of the recommendations contained in the following chapters of this report.

NOTES

1. Pope John Paul II, Address to the National Conference of the Italian Federation of Family Advisory Bureau of Christian Inspiration, March 28, 1987, *L'Osservatore Romano,* April 27, 1987.
2. *Economic Justice for All,* Pastoral Letter on Catholic Social Teaching and the U.S. Economy, Washington, DC, U.S. Catholic Conference, 1987, no. 122.
3. *Economic Justice for All,* no. 61.
4. *Economic Justice for All,* no. 80.
5. Pope John XXIII, *Christianity and Social Progress (Mater et Magistra),* 1961, no. 82-103; Pope John XXIII, *Peace on Earth, (Pacem in Terris),* 1963, no. 23-24; Pope John Paul II, *On HumanWork (Laborem Exercens),* 1981, no. 19-20.
6. *Economic Justice for All,* no. 100.

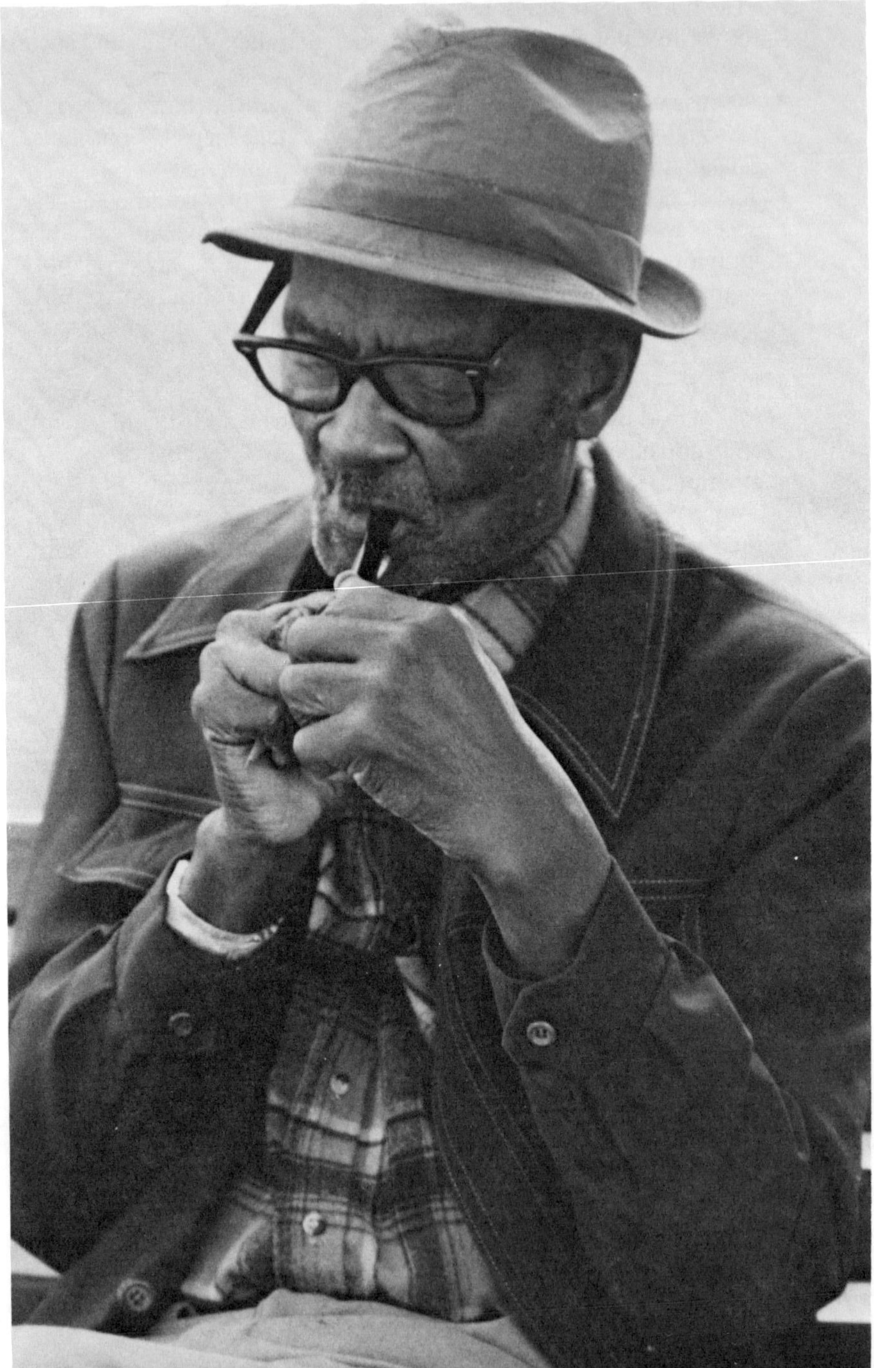

3

Responding to the Elderly-At-Risk

A Call to the Whole Church

To say that God cries out to persons in the circumstances and events of their lives is to recall that they are born and experience joy and pain, sickness and health, growth and decline, and finally death within families, parishes, and local communities. These words remind us that the life of the Church and the many expressions of its healthcare ministry are broader and more varied than their more visible institutional manifestations.

To say that God reveals himself in the midst of everyday occurrences reminds us also that health and healing from a Christian perspective mean wholeness that is not only physical and emotional, but also spiritual and social. Thus, the Catholic healthcare ministry is concerned about the health and well-being of persons in the context of their families and neighborhoods, as well as in hospitals and nursing care facilities.

A wholistic healthcare ministry is concerned about such factors as adequate food, clothing, and shelter, and it addresses public health measures such as immunization, safe drinking water, and adequate sanitation. This ministry reaches out through its various apostolates to chemically dependent and developmentally impaired persons, serves those with chronic illnesses such as the functionally impaired elderly, and seeks to support and comfort their families and caregivers.

Thus, Christians believe that health is more than a medical concern and that the restoration of health and maintenance of good health are not solely the responsibility of physicians, nurses, hospitals, and nursing care facilities. "We all bear a responsibility in this regard, both as individuals and as members of larger social and religious institutions."[1]

This broader understanding of the healthcare ministry has several important implications for the Church and its services to the frail elderly. First, Catholics cannot comfortably relegate the responsibility for health to the Church's hospitals and nursing care facilities. As important as acute, rehabilitative, and nursing care are to the spectrum of available long term care services, the dependent elderly and their families have needs that cannot be satisfied by these services alone. Parishes, Charities agencies, and dioceses are all intimately linked to the healthcare ministry.

Second, the entire Church must look for new ways of placing the enormous competence and commitment of its Catholic health facilities and diocesan Charities USA programs at the service of parish ministries to the elderly and their families. At the same time the network of parish ministers could certainly enrich the institutional healthcare ministry in areas such as pastoral visiting and recreational programming.

As noted earlier, long term care refers to a spectrum of services that includes institutions such as hospitals and nursing care facilities, as well as home care, respite and day care, hospice services, and special housing. Properly organized and managed, the services should be adjusted to the individual requirements of the frail elderly and allow for the easy transition from one program to another.

The Church has a rich array of formal health and social services provided by nearly 645 hospitals and 437 nursing homes. Virtually all diocesan Catholic Charities USA agencies in the United States provide services to the elderly, such as counseling (83 agencies serving 56,436 people), home care (26 agencies serving 11,000 people), health programs (34 agencies serving 34,000 people), and food programs (47 dioceses serving 320,000 people). However, perhaps as a reflection of the lack of coordination that characterizes long term care generally in the United States today, the Church's various services often relate awkwardly to each other. In this regard, hospital administrators, pastors, Charities USA directors, and representatives of health ministries that lie outside the Church's more formal institutionalized healthcare ministries need to communicate much more effectively with one another than they presently do.

Successful Church programs for frail elderly persons and their friends can be initiated when professionals involved in Catholic health and Charities USA begin asking how *together* they might develop answers to such questions as: How can we help the impaired elderly and their stressed caregivers by working with parishes to develop programs for them? Can we assist in the development of affinity and peer groups that give both knowledge and psychological support? Can we help parishes to ensure continuity of care for elderly persons discharged to their homes? Can we help the parish with adult day care, respite, and hospice programs?

Clearly the whole Church is called to place its many resources at the service of the frail elderly, especially those who are poor and alone. Clearly, too, the many elderly persons within the Church who are healthy and financially secure should see themselves as a potentially valuable resource in the Church's pastoral mission to those in need within their communities.

The Parish

Many Parishes Have a Growing Number of Elderly

Many parishes in the United States have large numbers of elderly members. Researchers at the Third Age Center of Fordham University have preliminary data showing that on the average, 26 percent of the members in any given parish are likely to be age 65 or older, slightly over twice the proportion of older persons to the general population.[2] Some parishes, particularly those in mature urban neighborhoods or in retirement communities, consist almost entirely of persons over age 65. This special group of parishioners presents a unique set of pastoral challenges to the Church. The Catholic Charities USA parish outreach programs represent one attempt to respond.

The Spirituality of the Elderly

The elderly have a spirituality marked by their being well along on their life journey. Parish ministry should recognize their need for support and guidance and at the same time create opportunities for them to share their mature faith experience with the community. The parish should be a place where the elderly are able to interpret their lives in the light of faith and, in doing so, have it confirmed by the community. The younger community members can draw strength and courage from the experience and example of the elderly members.

Contributions of the Elderly

Older persons who are retired and whose families are raised often may have time to give to parish activities. Typically, they also have skills and talents that can significantly enrich the life of the parish community. The pastor has a particular responsibility to call forth these persons who are able to put their time and talents to the service of the community. The invitation to serve does not always have to come from the pastor. The elderly themselves can encourage each other to participate by organizing programs that address a particular parish or community need. In contributing to the life of the parish, the elderly find that many of their own social and personal needs are met. Through prayer and redemptive suffering, the frail can continue to contribute to the vitality of the faith community.

Pastoral Care Staff

Family members, friends, and parishioners work along with the professionally trained and salaried pastoral care workers to offer spiritual support to the elderly. In a parish setting, pastoral visitors and Eucharistic ministers can be a vital link to the parish community for those who can no longer get to church. Their presence expresses the concern of the community for the person isolated by sickness or disability. They can often help the elderly person who feels alienated to be reconciled with God and with family members.

Professional pastoral care staffs have the educational background and professional experience to assume additional roles in the ministry to the elderly, such as spiritual direction, preparation of special prayer services, education of others in ministry to the elderly, and counseling of the elderly and their caregivers. Those who are ordained have the additional privilege and responsibility of enhancing the quality of life for the elderly through sacramental ministry.

Intentional Parish Plan for Ministry with the Elderly

Every parish, particularly those with many elderly members, should develop a pastoral plan with the participation of the elderly themselves. It should reflect a Christian perspective on the aging experience, with components that address spiritual growth, participation in the community through service, and continuing education in Christian moral responsibility.

The development of a useful plan presupposes a systematic assessment of the elderly's specific needs in the parish and surrounding community along with an assessment of the resources that can be called on to respond. These resources should include professionals from the pastoral, medical, social welfare, and education committees, as well as other volunteers from the parish community.

The plan should reflect the unique personality of the parish and its special needs and capabilities. Features that should be common to all plans would be (1) the elimination of barriers to participation in worship and parish activities (e.g., steps, poor acoustics, small print publications); (2) outreach to those who cannot come to church (e.g., home-delivered meals,

Communion, phone calls); and (3) support for family members who are the primary caregivers of the frail elderly (e.g., counseling, respite help, links to social service and healthcare agencies).

Care of the Frail Elderly

Intentional pastoral planning for the elderly at the parish level is particularly urgent because of the growing number of frail elderly living alone with very limited resources. They are dependent on their relatives, friends, and neighbors to provide their most vital needs. When they are provided that support, with perhaps regular visits of a home care nurse, they are able to remain at home in familiar surroundings.

It is in the lives of these persons that one particularly hears the call for compassion. The person in need may be someone who is alienated from relatives or is the lone survivor in the family. Parish volunteers who reach out to the elderly members of the community, especially those who live alone, and offer them meals, transportation, help with personal errands, or even a little conversation, are making visible the love of the invisible God.

Witness to Community and Solidarity

Well-planned programs of support for the frail elderly, especially those who are poor, can give important institutional witness to the values of community, collaboration, and solidarity with the most vulnerable. Churches that have been able to form communities of mutual service find their service strengthened, challenged, and mirrored in their sacramental life, particularly in their Eucharistic celebrations. The Eucharist often becomes what it is meant to be—a celebration of unity and loving, self-giving care for one another.

The Diocese

A Clear Call to Minister to the Elderly

What is needed in each diocese is a clear call to the Catholic community to reach out to the elderly in its midst and an intentional pastoral plan to give shape and direction to a coordinated diocesan response to that call. A major contribution can and should be made to this plan's development by persons over 65 who are able and willing to give their time and talent to the effort. Planning for ministry to the aged in this way should become integrated into the regular diocesan planning process. The special focus of pastoral planning for the elderly should be the frail elderly who are poor and living alone.

Encouraging Cooperation

Bishops have a particular leadership role to play in encouraging local efforts to coordinate formal and informal services for the elderly. In cases where Catholic healthcare providers and Catholic Charities are working in isolation from each other or at cross purposes, bishops may be able to convene them for collaborative planning and action. In areas where parishes or volunteer groups are looking for links with government programs, professional agencies, or healthcare providers, diocesan staff may be able to facilitate those connections. In a study of 925 Catholic parishes, 51 percent had some contact with Catholic social services, whereas only 11 percent had contact with nursing care facilities and 26 percent with hospitals.[3]

Programs to Support Parish Ministry

Some dioceses have resources to offer programs and services needed to support the direct ministry to the elderly occurring in parishes, neighborhoods, institutions, and housing complexes. The diocesan church has only rarely developed a vision and technique to address the full range of frail persons' needs with a recognition of the special opportunities at its disposal. The diocese can offer a variety of educational programs: biblical studies, theology and spirituality, pastoral formation, counseling, community organization, and group-process training. It can also provide retreats, respite, and support programs for the caregivers of the elderly. In an area where a pressing need for housing exists, the diocese may take on the development of group homes, residential care homes, or even larger congregate housing projects.[4]

The diocese should offer outreach programs to parishes to develop local parish leadership. Even when they are successful, parish networks of volunteers, as with other volunteer networks, can be fragile. They need to be buttressed by the type of institutional supports that social service agencies and healthcare facilities provide: case management services, home health programs, adult day care centers, hospice programs, and respite care programs for caregivers. Some of these programs and services are being offered in many communities under the auspices of the diocese through Catholic Charities USA or a coordinator of programs and services for the aging.

Public Awareness and Advocacy

Since the legislative and financial framework for the provision of services to the aging is set by governmental bodies at the federal, state, and local levels, the Church and the institutions under Catholic auspices have a vital role to play in public debates that help to reshape that currently fragmented framework. The influence that each of them is capable of exercising individually is likely to be enhanced by systematic efforts to work together. Moreover, collaboration in the public realm is a way to give concrete expression to the values of community and solidarity in the pursuit of the common good.

Some of this cooperative activity is possible at the local level in the form of community health education and enablement programming. Communication and, when opportune, concerted action are also needed at the state level. State legislatures have controlling influence over laws governing the rights of the frail elderly, licensing and regulating of nursing care facilities, Medicaid reimbursement, and the administration of the programs created by the Older Americans Act.

Access and Right to Healthcare

Government reimbursement programs are of interest to the Church because the amounts of government money available and the regulations governing eligibility directly affect the kinds of services that are available as well as persons' access to those services. Indirectly, these factors affect the quality of care that providers are able to offer those who do gain access.

Through its theologians and papal and episcopal statements, the Catholic Church insists that all persons have a right to healthcare. This right is predicated on the understanding that health is a prerequisite to the satisfaction of other basic human needs. A socioeconomic structure that makes available a high quality of care to some people, while others in the same society are deprived, calls for a redistribution of healthcare resources to ensure that all have access to what they need.[5]

Even as Church authorities and Catholic providers advocate more equitable government support for the care of the elderly with limited resources, they commit themselves to seeking philanthropic support and to putting a proportion of their own institutional resources at risk to ensure that persons are not denied access to the care they need.

Legislation on Advance Directives

The recent interest in "living will" legislation and proxy healthcare decision making reflects, in part, the worry that many elderly have about the prospect of being kept alive on life-support systems without their consent. Many are just as concerned that healthcare professionals may assume unjustifiably and without consulting them that they are "too old" or "too sick" to receive a certain treatment.

These legislative initiatives and the set of moral issues that such legislation attempts to address are of particular interest to the Church. The Catholic tradition looks on life as a gift of God that human beings hold in trust. Within this perspective, Church representatives have cautiously monitored and supported laws that protect persons' rights to participate in their treatment decisions and that provide a way for them to make their wishes known in advance should they become incompetent or permanently comatose at the end of life. Likewise, acting within this perspective, the Church has actively opposed legislation that purports to legitimize euthanasia or assisted suicide.[6]

Collaboration on Behalf of the Elderly-At-Risk

Catholics Working Together

This report has identified three factors that challenge the leadership of various Catholic ministries to reach out and to begin to collaborate with one another on behalf of the frail elderly and their caregivers. First, the percentage of Americans over age 65 is growing rapidly, and among them the fastest-growing percentage is the group over 85. Second, most care and support for the frail elderly occur outside of hospitals and nursing care facilities, and most of that is done by family and friends in stress-filled circumstances. Third, too many frail elderly are not receiving appropriate care because of our fragmented service delivery system and/or because they have no family, friends, or financial resources.

This situation calls for joint planning at all levels of institutional organization, collaboration among providers of services to coordinate the provision of an integrated set of services to the frail elderly and their families, and a coordinated effort to raise public awareness and urge financial support for the care of those at risk.

Collaboration with Others in Ministry and Advocacy

The Catholic Church is collaborating with a variety of other religious groups and healthcare and social agencies to enhance the scope and quality of ministry to the elderly in the community. Also, since it does not claim that its advocacy positions on behalf of human rights and respect for life are Catholic positions as such, it forms coalitions with other groups that share the same concern for protecting these values on behalf of the elderly.

Task Force Recommendations for the Whole Church

Parishes

- That parish programs for the elderly be developed consisting of the following components:
    1. Active support and encouragement by the pastor and parochial leadership
    2. Assessment of the needs and available resources, including parish demographics, transportation and housing needs, physical plan (acoustics, barriers, available space for programs), special needs, pool of expertise/skills among the elderly, and community agencies and services
    3. *Intentional* pastoral plan for the elderly that addresses the spirituality, service potential, and value commitments of the elderly, with participation by elderly parishioners in the plan's development

4. Individual assigned or identified to coordinate a program
5. An established evaluation group, including elderly parishioners, with whom program coordinator meets regularly for program assessment and planning
6. Budget sufficient to support programs
7. Program of formation in ministry that includes ongoing support along with initial formation
8. Organizational links to available consultation and support from the diocese, social service agencies, healthcare providers, and individual professions
9. Outreach to other Church and neighborhood groups

- That parishes, in collaboration with long term care administrators and diocesan staff, develop pastoral plans for ministry in nursing care facilities and various other settings, such as day care centers and housing complexes; such plans should create opportunities for laypersons to serve as ministers to the frail elderly
- That Catholic ministers, laypersons, and clergy take advantage of opportunities for interfaith and interagency cooperation in appropriate areas of ministry to the elderly

Dioceses

- That diocesan leadership, such as diocesan commissions, pastoral letters, or major initiatives in pastoral planning, articulate more clearly and forcefully the call to minister to the frail elderly
- That ministry to and with the elderly be brought into the mainstream of diocesan pastoral planning
- That diocesan leadership advocate the coordination of formal (healthcare and social services) and informal (parish and neighborhood support) services for the elderly at the local level
- That dioceses facilitate parish ministry to older persons by making available pastoral formation and educational programs, community organization training, and respite and support programs for caregivers, as well as seed money and recognition
- That diocesan staff help to link parishes with community resources, e.g., healthcare facilities, Charities agencies, social service agencies, colleges and universities, and area agencies on aging
- That dioceses advocates through Catholic Charities or other agencies, the development of those direct services that address the most urgent needs not being met locally, e.g., housing, respite care, counseling, educational and cultural programming, retreats, coordination of information, and referral services

State Catholic Conferences

- That state Catholic conferences maintain an active public advocacy posture on behalf of the frail elderly
- That conferences assume an advocacy posture in state legislative activity regarding such issues as protecting the rights of the frail elderly, housing, licensing and regulating healthcare services, reimbursement, advance directives such as "living wills," and state support for Older Americans Act programs
- That staffs of Catholic conferences be well educated and formed in the theological and ethical tradition of the Church as it relates to these issues
- That state Catholic conferences work with their federal legislators to advocate the federal policy reforms identified in Chapter 5

National Catholic Organizations

- That National Conference of Catholic Bishops (NCCB)/U.S. Catholic Conference (USCC), The Catholic Health Association of the United States (CHA), and Catholic Charities USA advocate a pastorally oriented understanding of aging in our society that draws on the Catholic faith tradition. This understanding, because it is meant to have a broad pastoral influence, should be easily understood by a general audience. "Respect Life Week" could provide the occasion for a jointly sponsored initiative to raise awareness about the frail elderly.
- That NCCB/USCC, CHA, and Catholic Charities USA convene a group of individuals responsible for pastoral care in national pastoral associations to develop a set of standards and credentials for conducting pastoral care programs in long term care. American Association of Homes for the Aging (AAHA), American Association of Retired Persons (AARP), and American Health Care Association (AHCA) should also be represented.
- That Catholic Charities USA agencies, in coordination with parish ministries to the poor, work to identify persons eligible for, but not yet enrolled in, state Medicaid programs.

NOTES

1. "Health and Health Care: A Pastoral Letter of the American Catholic Bishops," Washington, DC, U.S. Catholic Conference, Nov. 19, 1981, p. 6.
2. New York State Catholic Conference Commission on the Elderly, Albany, NY, Fall 1985, p. 5.
3. New York State Catholic Conference, p. 12.
4. Constance Clark, *Serving Older Persons,* 3rd ed., Commission on Aging, Washington, DC, Catholic Charities USA, 1987.
5. Pope John XXIII, *Peace on Earth,* 1963; Pope Paul VI, *Development of Peoples,* 1967; U.S. Bishops' Pastoral, "Economic Justice for All," 1986.

6. Vatican Declaration on Euthanasia, 1980; "Commentary on the Uniform Act for the Rights of the Terminally Ill," Committee for Pro-Life Activities of the National Conference of Catholic Bishops; "A Proposal for Assisted Suicide," *CACH Networking,* California Association of Catholic Hospitals, vol. 16, Winter, 1988; "Christian Affirmation of Life," St. Louis, The Catholic Health Association of the United States, 1987; J. Stuart Showalter and Brian Andrew, *To Treat or Not to Treat,* St. Louis, The Catholic Health Association of the United States, 1984.

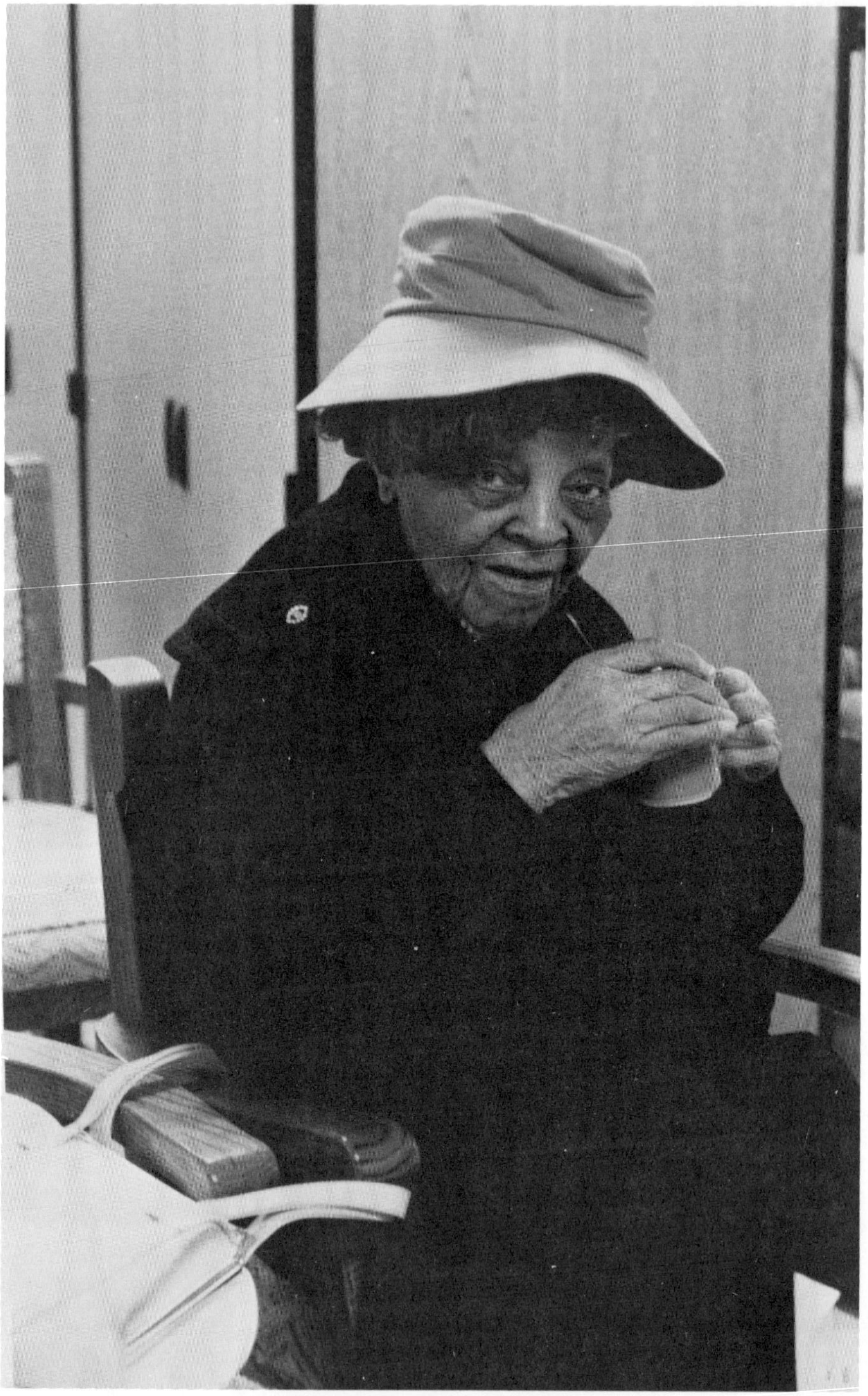

4

A Call to the Institutional Catholic Health-care Ministry

In recent years, many Catholic healthcare organizations and systems have been expanding their long term and continuing care services by acquiring nursing care facilities, adult day care programs, home health services, retirement housing, and a variety of other services.

While many of these services were started in response to perceived community needs, others were initiated in response to the intensely competitive market environments in which most healthcare organizations find themselves today. Price competition, government cutbacks, and commercialization have made even not-for-profit institutions increasingly preoccupied with the business environment, market plans, market penetration, and outreach programs that attract patients who pay well.

For instance, some Catholic and other healthcare organizations have developed vertically integrated models of service acquisition to improve their hospitals' market positions by providing a variety of services that will attract elderly patients. (See Figure 1.) It is important to note that while many of these arrangements provide a wide array of integrated services, the integration is limited and is primarily from the acute facility's fiscal and management perspective, rather than from the clients' need perspective. Figure 2 illustrates how the same set of services, which are integrated from the hospital's perspective, might appear as separate and distinct to the elderly. Nevertheless, some healthcare organizations refer to a vertically integrated system or similar arrangement as a "continuum."

FIGURE 1

Vertically Integrated Model of Service Acquisition

Vertically Integrated Services

Acute Hospital

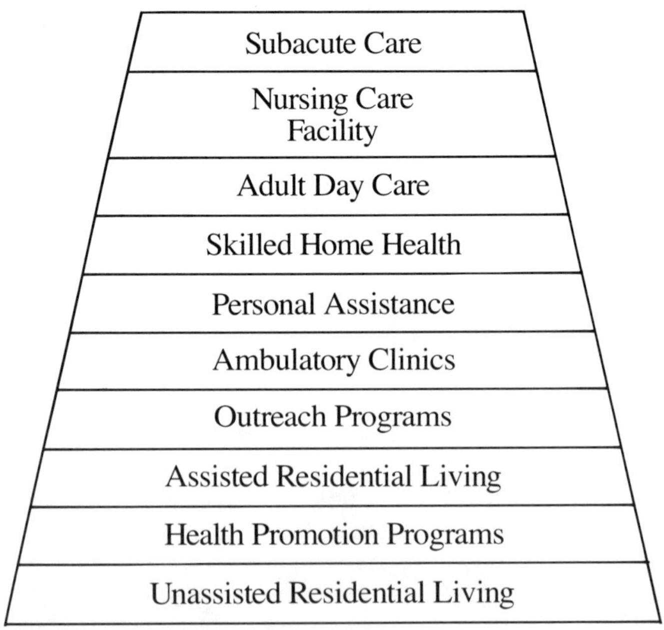
Subacute Care
Nursing Care Facility
Adult Day Care
Skilled Home Health
Personal Assistance
Ambulatory Clinics
Outreach Programs
Assisted Residential Living
Health Promotion Programs
Unassisted Residential Living

FIGURE 2

**System Development
from the Client's Perspective**

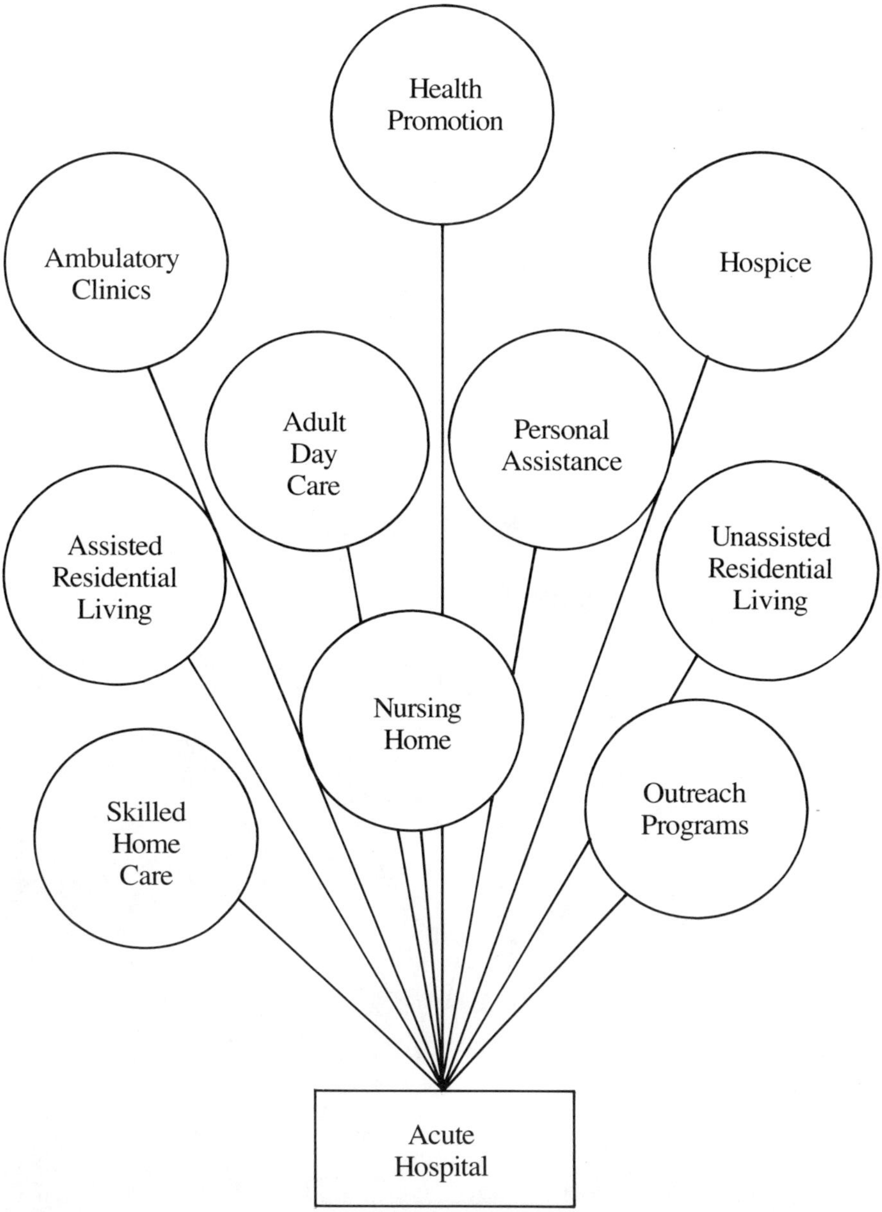

FIGURE 3

Unprofitable Services in Market-Driven Model

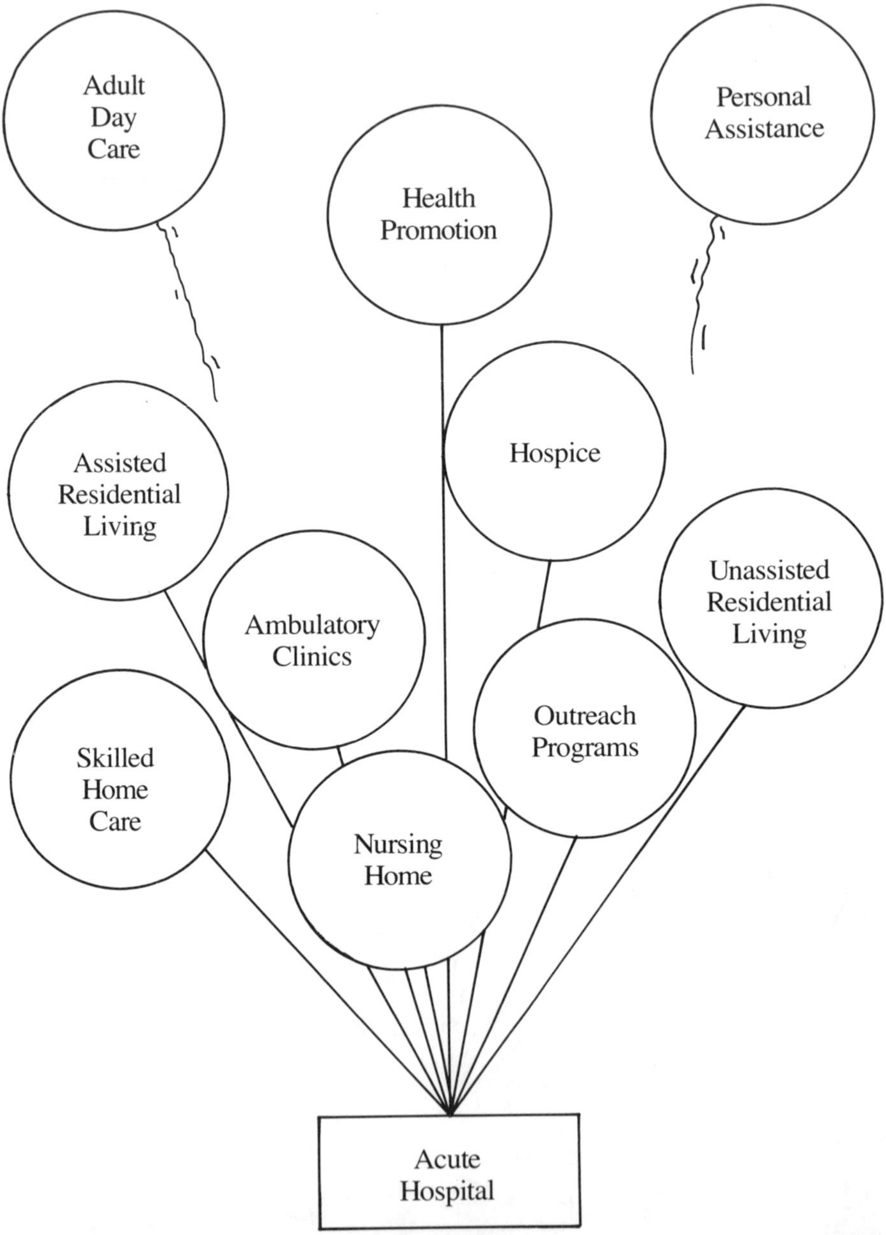

An explicit market focus may financially strengthen the healthcare organization and make a large array of services available to the community, but the result is not likely to be a continuum of care, since a true continuum is more than a collection of services related to the same institution.

As Chapter 1 emphasized, several other features are required. The first and most important is an explicit focus on the client's range of functional needs, as opposed to a primarily market-driven orientation.

The distinction is a critical one because the healthcare organization's strategic focus largely determines the *kinds* of services it develops for the frail elderly, the *degree* of internal service integration it implements, and the *role* it plays in the larger community to ensure that its own services are complemented by and integrated with other necessary supports. If the healthcare organization's primary departure point is a market focus, then it will acquire services based primarily on what they can do to strengthen the organization. In a market-driven model, services that turn out to be financial losers may be let go. (See Figure 3.)

On the other hand, a client-focused healthcare organization first determines what services it must provide, or arrange to be provided by others, in order to ensure that the frail elderly and their caregivers receive an appropriate mix of formal and informal supports as they move from one functional state to another.

The range of available services in a client-focused continuum of care will be comprehensive and cover the spectrum from social-intensive, community based, primarily outpatient care to health intensive, institution based, primarily inpatient care. Not all the services provided by the healthcare organization or by other providers in the larger continuum will be profitable. In fact, many providers are currently struggling to maintain some of their services to the elderly. All the providers together will have to determine how the unprofitable-but-necessary services will be supported.

Second, the client-focused healthcare organization will make certain that its own departments are well integrated from the client's perspective, e.g., do the hospital outpatient services departments know about and work with the hospital-sponsored hospice program?

Third, the client-focused healthcare organization will facilitate the provision of the community leadership necessary to guarantee that the essential integrating elements described in Chapter 1 are developed and maintained (planning, care management, information systems, financing, administrative structure). These will ensure that the continuum remains focused on the client and avoids competing and duplicative programs, communication gaps, and budget conflicts.

Ernestine's case (see Introduction) highlights the significant differences that exist between the market-oriented and client-focused approaches to service delivery. To satisfy her desire to remain as independent as possible and stay in her own home, she will require a wide variety of integrated medical and social services. Unfortunately, and as Chapter 1 noted, while she is known to a number of health and social service providers, none of them has or is able to take responsibility for organizing and monitoring a program of care for her.

This fact will have severe consequences for Ernestine. As her heart ailment and diabetes worsen, her dysfunction will increase with respect to her need for personal care services. Thus, her reliance on neighbors and community supports will increase. If those supports (home health, personal care services, transportation to and from her physician's office, etc.) are unavailable or not properly coordinated for Ernestine, she will be admitted to a nursing care facility, not necessarily because of any demonstrated need for institutionally provided skilled nursing services, but because "there's nowhere else to go."

Ernestine is not unique. Her situation and those of the many others like her exemplify the need for fundamental system-wide reform. The way the nation's current long term care system both fails and manipulates the frail elderly is too often an affront to human dignity.

Catholic healthcare organizations are places of enormous competence and commitment. As such, they are a moral force in the communities they serve and can be agents for improving the common good. In this regard, the concept of a continuum of care offers Catholic healthcare organizations a way to ameliorate the harsher aspects of the current long term care system by making it work better for the functionally impaired elderly. Properly implemented, a continuum of care will better identify the frail elderly needs and make available a wider spectrum of services than otherwise would be available. Together, all these things challenge Catholic healthcare facilities in several important ways.

Catholic healthcare organizations located in communities in which a continuum of care does not presently exist should consider providing the leadership necessary to organizing one. In communities where a continuum of care already exists or is being planned, Catholic healthcare organizations should consider how they might become an active participant. And each Catholic healthcare facility should consider how an explicit client focus might help it better complement and integrate its own service mix.

For the Church, a "successful" healthcare organization is characterized by more than its productive efficiency or the amount of quality healthcare it provides. The Church also wants to know how the institution responds to people's special needs. "The dignity of the human person, realized in community with others, is the criterion against which all aspects of economic life must be measured."[1] A profound concern for and energetic response to the needs of the frail elderly must then become a priority in the Catholic institution's planning and budgeting process. The fundamental norm is this: What is happening to the frail elderly as a result of this action? This is not the only and may not always be the most important question, but it is essential if the organization is to address the service of the functionally impaired elderly.

Assets and Challenges

The Task Force does not underestimate the considerable difficulty involved in integrating the concepts and principles articulated in this report into the daily practice of a complex healthcare organization. In addition to the obstacles to a continuum of care identified in Chapter 1, private and public program cost controls coupled with intensive price competition place today's healthcare organizations under enormous pressure.

This report neither discounts nor minimizes the operational demands these pressures place on not-for-profit healthcare facilities' management. In such an environment it is a difficult and delicate task to balance a voluntary institution's responsibility to serve its community with its concomitant duty to preserve its assets so that it will survive to meet future community needs.

In fact, the Task Force believes that today's free market, pro-competition policy orientation too often disrupts this balance by pressuring some voluntary healthcare facilities into emphasizing concerns related to institutional fiscal strength and market position to the diminishment of their important, indeed primary, noneconomic objectives.

Some institutions justify their business emphasis by reference to the formulation "no margin, no mission." But this approach is not appropriate to the not-for-profit setting since it makes an institution's mission the handmaiden of its necessary business imperatives. A more appropriate, though more challenging, practice followed by many voluntary healthcare facilities is to identify the institution's mission and then determine how to assemble the public, private, and charitable resources necessary to implement it and maintain it over time.

The method recognizes the primacy of mission without disparaging the legitimate role of sound business practices in the operation of a voluntary healthcare facility. It also accords favorably with the religious origins of Catholic healthcare institutions; most of which were started in response to community need and sustained in faith often under difficult circumstances and at considerable personal, material, and financial sacrifice.

The "client's wholistic needs first" vision articulated in this report represents a fundamental challenge to today's over-reliance on price competition in the delivery of healthcare and the commercialized message it elicits about building a "hospital flagship" arrangement of services. It also challenges Catholic healthcare leaders to look up and out of the trenches and in a spirit of solidarity to identify with their facility's elderly clients who may be even more adversely affected by the problems associated with our fragmented healthcare system.

However, the Task Force would also ask Catholic healthcare organizations to consider that a clear focus on client need in the context of the organization's mission may be an aid, not a hindrance, to the institution's survival in these difficult times. A clarification of institutional values creates criteria that can free healthcare organization managers to make critical choices about the institution's operational direction and help them resist questionable actions for a quick fix.

A clear emphasis on client-focused care and community service can build valuable community and, therefore, political support for the healthcare organization in an era of budget-driven public program cost reductions. It will also reinforce and legitimize the healthcare organization's community service role at a time when many local, state, and federal policy makers are questioning whether or not not-for-profit healthcare organizations are any longer entitled to tax-exempt status.

Finally, the inclusion of a client-focused continuum of care in a healthcare organization's strategic plan and operations may position the organization to become the "provider of choice" for private and public insurers. These insurers are and increasingly will be seeking to contract with providers who can offer their beneficiaries a wide range of appropriate, integrated, and cost-effective services.

In summary, for Catholic healthcare organizations to influence the delivery and management of services for the elderly-at-risk, their leadership must recognize the need to change the focus of healthcare delivery from an episodic, acute-disease crisis orientation to a multilevel, integrated array of services that is responsive to patient needs and emphasizes prevention and rehabilitation. This requires management to change from a product-line orientation to a focus that is built on the client's total needs. It involves collaboration with Catholic and other providers and community and neighborhood organizations. Catholic healthcare providers, parishes, Charities agencies, and universities can have a great influence on creating a system within their communities. Building on what is already present and learning from others will expedite the development of a continuum of care that is responsive to the elderly-at-risk and their caregivers' needs.

Recommendations to the Institutional Catholic Healthcare Ministry

Religious Institutes Who Sponsor Healthcare Organizations

- That they identify the frail elderly population as a focus of their own ministry in the healthcare setting
- That they provide the inspiration, the commitment, and the leadership for serving the frail elderly. They can recognize and support the continuum where it is already in place and facilitate the implementation of the integrating elements in their healthcare ministries where it does not exist.

- That sponsoring religious orders educate themselves about the continuum of care as it may pertain to the long term needs of their own frail elderly members
- That they consider "recycling" their unused institute-owned space and facilities for health and other purposes to respond to the needs of the frail elderly in the community
- That homes for retired religious consider making some of their services and activities available to the frail elderly in the community as a further extension of the religious' ministry

Systems Leadership

- That the leadership of Catholic healthcare systems include the continuum of care in their strategic planning and budgeting processes, recognizing that this will be an incremental process
- That they seek to consult and hire professionals with specific knowledge and expertise in the care of the elderly
- That they foster collaboration among healthcare providers with the goal of participation in the continuum of care to serve the client foremost. Collaboration should also be sought with parishes, interfaith groups, Catholic Charities, and community groups and agencies.

Catholic Healthcare Providers

- That Catholic healthcare providers promote a community assessment to include evaluation of the frail elderly's needs and available services and develop a strategic plan that includes a continuum of care. Providers of Catholic healthcare may initiate the assessment themselves or cooperate with other facilities and agencies within the community who are also interested in the continuum.
- That in developing their strategies for a continuum of care, they premise their efforts on the needs of persons or communities (as contrasted with service/program availability). They then should recognize and establish relationships with existing programs and services that are part of such strategies or could be affected by their development.
- That acute care organizations examine their own policies and performance in relation to the unique needs of the frail elderly. Even during the acute phase of an illness, most elderly have compelling long term healthcare needs (e.g., to remain as independent as possible, to be mobile and oriented). The type and quality of acute care received by the frail elderly can have an enormous potential to affect functioning for better or worse.

- That they provide and/or encourage the leadership that will help establish programs and services for the elderly-at-risk within their respective parishes and other local community group settings
- That they collaborate with local churches, Catholic Charities, and dioceses to promote mechanisms to help parishes establish ministries that support, educate, encourage, and offer respite for informal and family caregivers
- That they review their public relations activities for the image of aging being projected by the organization. They should actively participate in community relations and programming that enhance respect for older adults and the inherent dignity of each person.
- That they include the funding of progressive changes to develop a true continuum of care in each year's budget development process
- That they include progressive changes toward a continuum of care in the CEO's performance evaluation goals
- That they provide training of all employees on the aging process, hospitality and guest relations for older adults, all health and community services available for the older adult, referral routes, and key persons to access these services
- That they assertively advocate a more rational long term care delivery system. They should consider legislative positions in light of the older adult's needs, as well as the organization's business position.

Catholic Health Association

- That CHA develop educational programs for the healthcare ministry regarding interdisciplinary continuum of care strategies. These programs could be used by providers to identify the issues and develop the long-range strategy for participating in a continuum of care.
- That CHA exercise and foster leadership in the area of long term care of the frail elderly by collaborating with other appropriate national and state organizations. This will ensure that its understanding of the necessity for interdisciplinary continuum of care strategies animates public policy and private-sector decision making.
- That CHA consider the possibility of offering long term care insurance to its employees
- That CHA identify and/or facilitate the development of models for:
  1. Continuum of care strategies
  2. Supporting and educating professional caregivers
- That CHA continue its advocacy of federal legislative and regulatory improvements in access for the elderly, particularly the

elderly-at-risk, to essential social—including health—programs and services (Medicare, long term care insurance, etc.)

- That CHA identify expert gerontologists for the purpose of referral to healthcare providers who are contemplating or developing strategies for a continuum of care
- That CHA encourage appropriate universities to expand their professional offerings relative to geriatric-specific programming. CHA should also encourage Catholic healthcare organizations to use geriatric specialists to assist in the development, implementation, and evaluation of programs and services for the elderly-at-risk.

NOTE

1. "Catholic Social Teaching and the U.S. Economy," no. 150, *Origins* 14:22/23, Nov. 15, 1984.

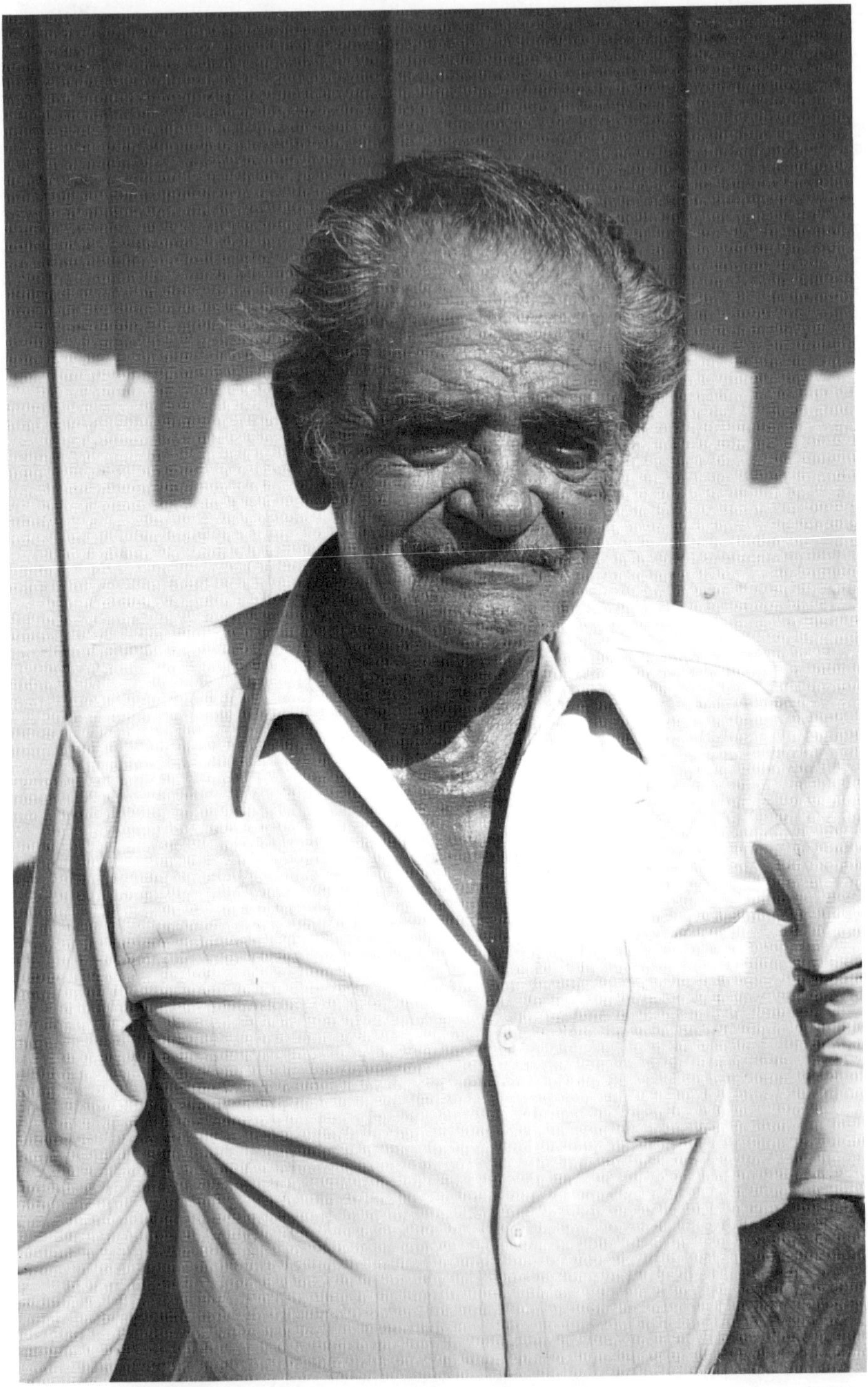

5

The Elderly-At-Risk and the Role of Government

No national policy exists on the long term care needs of the frail elderly. Although the United States has a variety of distinct programs that address particular problems faced by the elderly-at-risk—illness, lack of adequate nutrition, isolation, frailty, lack of income—the nation does not have a common vision as to how these services might be supplemented, integrated, and generally much better coordinated in each community and rural area.

As noted in earlier chapters of this report, some problems of the elderly are defined by reimbursement biases and institutional frameworks as health problems, but these are actually problems of housing and social service delivery. For example, many persons currently reside in nursing care facilities because of a lack of any viable housing alternative supplemented by social support such as meals and assistance with daily living.

Some of these elderly could be well assisted by targeting services to persons in their own homes, which could prevent premature institutionalization. Medicaid cutbacks in nursing care facility services must be redressed by alternative housing and social service arrangements. Housing services provided by the Department of Housing and Urban Development (HUD) are sometimes viewed as an alternative but are inappropriate, since elderly persons must be ambulatory to qualify.

The reimbursement systems under Medicare and Medicaid have fueled the fragmented nature of services by virtue of their payment for services rather than for coordinated care. For example, patients being discharged from the hospital may find themselves without support in their homes or communities to meet basic needs. More extensive rehabilitation, home health services, and social services are required in a coordinated fashion so as not to jeopardize the quality of life of elderly persons. However, public policy must strike a balance in offering home care services to those who require them without substituting for the family-provided care where it is already in place.

Another concern is that current reimbursement policies may preclude the appropriate diagnostic, therapeutic, and rehabilitative care that some elderly persons need. Indeed, the incidence and prevalence of mental illness increases with age, but reimbursement policies are geared toward acute physical illness rather than mental illness. Thus, an appropriate mix of services is needed to meet the essential needs of the frail elderly.

Continuing care communities are one example of attempts to provide some elderly persons with coordinated housing, health, and social services. This option, however, is available only to those elderly with the financial means to afford such accommodations. To serve as a possible alternative for the less affluent elderly, the need exists to reduce the cost of continuing care communities.

As noted in Chapter 1, several demonstration projects authorized under Medicaid waivers suggest that important changes in the way long term care services are coordinated and integrated can be accomplished in a cost-effective manner and can make a positive difference in the lives of the frail elderly. They also offer the hope that comprehensive policy reform will someday allow each U.S. community to develop its own continuum of care.

The Task Force believes that this will not occur, however, until the nation develops a social insurance program whereby a defined degree of disability would trigger eligibility for a variety of services in one's home, in a social institution such as a home for the aging that provides housing and social services, or in an institution that provides needed medical care.

Our long-range vision of comprehensive and coordinated health and social services for the elderly will require a comprehensive and coordinated legislative effort. The Task Force recognizes that policy reform in the United States is rarely comprehensive. It also recognizes the political restraint attendant on the large federal deficits created by existing programs.

This report, therefore, will focus on suggestions for incremental legislative reforms to move the "system" in the right direction. The Task Force wishes to emphasize, however, that the typically American penchant for incremental change cannot long conceal the requirement for fundamental long term care policy reform. This is a goal toward which we should all be working.

The following sections examine the strengths and weaknesses of existing public programs as well as future and private options for meeting the health, housing, and income needs of the elderly. Recommendations are made for improvements in existing government programs. The policy focus is on the years until 2000.

Medicare

Medicare is the companion healthcare program for Social Security enacted into law in 1965 under Title XVIII of the Social Security Act. Medicare helps pay the healthcare of the elderly and, under certain conditions, of permanently disabled persons under 65 and of individuals with end-stage renal disease. In fiscal year 1985, $61 billion was paid for the healthcare of the 27 million elderly persons enrolled in the program.

Medicare consists of two parts: the Hospital Insurance (Part A) benefits and the Supplementary Medical Insurance (Part B) benefits. Part A is financed primarily through a payroll tax. As of 1988, 1.45 percent of an employee's earnings up to $45,000 are paid into the Hospital Insurance Trust Fund. An equivalent amount is matched by the employer. Part A covers acute inpatient hospital costs and hospice services. The Part B program covers physician visits and selected other outpatient services. It is financed by a combination of monthly premiums from Medicare beneficiaries and from general revenues. The Medicare Part B premium for 1988 is $24.80 per month.

According to the 1988 annual report of the Medicare Board of Trustees, the Hospital Insurance portion of Medicare should remain solvent until 2005 under current policies and moderate economic assumptions.[1] However, the trustees expressed concern about the rapid growth of Part B outlays, which have doubled in the last five years.

Strengths and Weaknesses

Medicare covers only a portion of the healthcare expenses of the elderly. Many elderly, especially the poor elderly, must bear medical expenses that amount to a significant portion of their incomes. Medicare covers the costs associated with acute care and hospice care. Extended care services in nursing care facilities and hospitals are included, but the conditions of coverage are very narrow and limited. Moreover, with the advent of prospective payment, physicians have incentive to discharge patients from acute hospitals sooner. Thus, patients may not be well equipped to care for themselves soon after an acute episode of illness. Very little research has been done relating to the impact of the new payment system on beneficiaries.

For example, the Medicare nursing care benefit covers only short term, post-acute care for persons needing skilled nursing or rehabilitative services. The Medicare nursing care and hospice benefits set specific and stringent requirements for the levels of skilled care or types of service allowed for Medicare coverage.

Since the home health benefit under Medicare is designed to be part of the continuum of care for an episode of acute illness, it is generally unavailable for long term needs that persist over time. Passage of the Omnibus Reconciliation Act in 1981 expanded the home health benefit by removing the limit on the number of covered home health visits, eliminating the requirement for a prior hospital stay, eliminating the deductible, and allowing more proprietary home health agencies to participate in the Medicare program.

One general concern about the Medicare program is that reimbursement for designated services is not responsive to the varying long term needs of the elderly.

Task Force Recommendations

- *Ensure Financial Solvency.* The financial solvency of Medicare has two components: ensuring adequate funding of the program and ensuring that those funds are appropriately used. Fiscal arguments can be made against Medicare expansions unless they are fully financed by users or through general revenues. Although a need exists to ensure greater protection for the elderly, the need also exists to remedy the problem of Medicare's current inadequate financing while acknowledging that the federal budget deficit is increasing.
- *Examine Cost Sharing.* The most often heard argument favoring increased cost sharing is that it presumably discourages unnecessary care. Conversely, those opposed argue that increased cost sharing would target precisely those beneficiaries who already have the greatest financial liabilities. Moreover, the Medicare program's present cost sharing does not account for the income of the elderly person. This is particularly a problem for low-income beneficiaries because state Medicaid programs now cover only 36 percent of the elderly living in poverty.

  This concern should be redressed by linking increases in out-of-pocket payments to ability to pay. This process is a complex one administratively but not impossible. There could be a philosophical problem with basing out-of-pocket expenses on the ability to pay because it potentially undermines the "earned right" to Medicare, by virtue of payments made during the working life. The income tax system could be used as a way to relate increased Medicare premiums to income. The insurance value of Part A could be taxed, along with the subsidized portion of Part B (that portion paid through general revenues).

These measures have the potential to generate Medicare savings of about $8 billion in 1990, which could be used to increase benefits and coverage for the poor elderly or to ensure solvency of the Medicare trust fund further into the future.

This approach of "income relating" Medicare premiums (i.e., structuring the *cost* of premiums according to ability to pay) is far superior to any attempt to "means test" the program (whereby *eligibility* for Medicare would be based on income). Medicare should be available to all persons over age 65.

- *Implement Catastrophic Healthcare Protection*. The recent catastrophic healthcare bill redresses some of the gaps in coverage for the elderly. The expansion of coverage to include prescription drugs is a positive step that will benefit many elderly persons. A cap on out-of-pocket expenses is also an important step. Because prior Medicare coverage paid slightly less than half of the elderly population's health expenses, potential benefit reforms may be very costly. The Medicare catastrophic legislation also authorizes $1.5 million for the establishment of a bipartisan commission on comprehensive healthcare. Among other duties, the commission is to make specific recommendations to Congress on measures to ensure availability of comprehensive long term care for Medicare beneficiaries.
- *Increase Home Health and Nursing Home Benefits*. Rehabilitative care and other services for post-acute care are an important but strictly limited component of Medicare coverage. These Medicare benefits should be expanded; currently Medicaid covers nursing home stays by default. Medicare should take care of all elderly healthcare, not just those resulting from acute episodes of illness.

Social Security

Social Security is the largest federal benefit program, accounting for more than one-half of all spending on the elderly. It provides monthly partial income replacement benefits to retired workers and their dependents and to survivors of insured workers. What is typically called Social Security is actually two separate insurance funds: Old Age and Survivors Insurance (OASI) and Disability Insurance (DI).

Contributions based on wage and salary workers' earnings up to a statutory maximum taxable amount each year are withheld and matched by employers. Employers and workers in 1988 each contribute 7.51 percent of the first $45,000 of an employee's salary. Self-employed individuals contribute 15.02 percent.

In 1985, more than 24 million people, or almost 1 of 7 persons, received Social Security benefits from the OASI program. This includes 22.4 million retired workers and 10.7 million spouses, children, and survivors. More than 90 percent of the elderly currently receive Social Security benefits.[2]

Strengths and Weaknesses

Social Security has been the major factor in improving the financial situation of the elderly. Over the past 15 years, the elderly as a group have moved from a position of being substantially poorer than the nonelderly to being at least as well off. The change resulted from cost of living adjustments in Social Security, as well as higher pensions and better returns on assets. The income increase occurred despite a substantial reduction in work-related earnings among the elderly. These gains have led to both a rapid growth in the ranks of the financially secure elderly and a rapid decline in the prevalence of poverty among the aged.

In addition to the remaining sizable group of poor elderly, a very large and growing concentration of elderly falls into the category of not poor but not financially secure, with incomes above the poverty level but below the mean. These elderly are still vulnerable to the financial stress attendant to the death of a spouse, loss of earning ability, slow erosion of resources because of extended longevity, or major medical expenses. Although the elderly should continue to share in general economic growth, standards of living are likely to increase at a slower pace for the less affluent elderly because they are more dependent on public sources of income.

Of particular concern are widows who are not eligible to receive Social Security benefits before age 60 unless they are caring for a dependent child. This is sometimes referred to as the "widow's gap," i.e., the years before age 60 when a widow without children under age 18 is not eligible for any survivor benefits. In addition, elderly widows are among the poorest elderly; in 1984, nearly one half of all poor elderly Social Security beneficiaries were widows.

Task Force Recommendations

- *Improve Benefits for Women*. The relative status of women, who are most vulnerable to poverty, could be improved under Social Security. This would have a positive impact on the income of women when they retire or are widowed.

- *Maintain Fiscal Soundness*. In contrast to Medicare, the Social Security OASDI (Old Age, Survivors, and Disability Insurance) trust funds are not in danger of financial insolvency. Indeed, reserves will increase significantly over the next several decades. It is important for our future that the reserves are maintained, rather than used to fund deficits, as in the Medicare trust fund.
- *Increase the Age of Eligibility for Benefits*. The age of retirement set at age 65 dates from the late 19th century. Because of the increased longevity of the elderly and their better health status and income, the Task Force supports the current policy of raising the age of eligibility for full benefits from 65 to 67. We would not object to looking into increasing the age of eligibility beyond 67. Further raising the retirement age now to take effect when the baby boomers start to retire in 25 years is a powerful means of keeping Social Security solvent in two ways: it would pay out to 20 to 25 percent fewer pensioners, and it would collect payroll taxes from 5 to 10 percent more workers.

Medicaid

Many elderly poor have their healthcare financed by Medicaid. Medicaid is the second largest government healthcare program after Medicare. Although Medicare is the primary source of healthcare for elderly Americans, Medicaid is important because it pays for the healthcare of many poor elderly and many elderly in nursing homes.

Medicaid was enacted into law under Title XIX of the Social Security Act and became effective on July 1, 1966. It succeeded earlier welfare-linked medical care programs, most notably the Kerr-Mills program of medical assistance for the aged.

Medicaid is administered by the states under broad federal requirements and guidelines, and rules and regulations vary considerably among states. Expenditures are paid from both federal and state funds. Federal funds account for approximately 55 percent of Medicaid expenditures. The exact state share varies by state and ranges from 50 percent to 77.4 percent.

Medicaid does not pay for the healthcare of all poor persons. It was intended to serve as a companion healthcare program for persons receiving cash assistance under the two major welfare programs: Supplemental Security Income (SSI) and Aid to Families with Dependent Children (AFDC). Ordinarily, receipt of a welfare payment through AFDC or SSI guarantees Medicaid eligibility. However, states may choose to use more stringent eligibility rules if they have followed them since before the inception of SSI in 1974.

Although the elderly constitute only 15 percent of those entitled to Medicaid, they account for almost 40 percent of Medicaid expenditures.[3]

This is primarily because the elderly are more likely to be in nursing homes. Such care is expensive and accounted nationally for approximately 46 percent of all Medicaid expenditures in 1986. About half of the elderly in nursing homes became eligible for Medicaid by spending down, i.e., incurring medical bills large enough to bring their incomes down to specified low eligibility levels.

Strengths and Weaknesses

One of the major weaknesses of the Medicaid program is that many elderly persons' out-of-pocket expenditures for healthcare constitute a substantial portion of their income. Many elderly poor are not covered by Medicaid, and not all healthcare expenses are publicly paid for under Medicare and Medicaid. As incomes rise, the proportion of persons making out-of-pocket healthcare expenditures that amount to 10 percent or more of their incomes falls sharply. Approximately 12 percent of the poor and near-poor spent 15 percent or more of their income on healthcare in 1980. Consequently, paying for out-of-pocket expenses is likely to strain the already tight budgets of low-income senior citizens or will push their out-of-pocket outlays so high as to deny them effective access to our healthcare system.

In regard to Medicaid, any practical strategy to provide appropriate care to elderly persons must examine the possibilities and limits of public-sector financing. Enormous social costs of caring for elderly persons cannot be absorbed by the federal and state governments alone. The resources of the elderly and the extent to which they themselves can pay for at least a portion of their care is an important consideration in deliberating public policy.

We view this as crucial in an attempt to ensure that public resources are used to assist the most vulnerable elderly—those without family or financial resources. Thus, strategies must focus particularly on the poor elderly, who are least able to afford care and who are most likely to need it, noting that the poor are generally in worse health than higher-income persons. Also, protective measures should be taken to avoid the devastating effects of major health expenses on even higher-income elderly.

Recommendations

- *Expand Medicaid Eligibility.* An expansion of Medicaid eligibility would be an appropriate policy change. The Omnibus Budget Reconciliation Act of 1986 allows states the option to extend Medicaid benefits to the elderly who have incomes above the SSI eligibility cutoff but are still below the federal poverty line. States can set the income thresholds at any level they choose, up to federal poverty levels. Although this measure is a major step forward, the next necessary step is to *require* states to offer

Medicaid benefits to the elderly with incomes between the SSI cutoff and the poverty level.

- *Expand Medicaid Benefits*. Home health benefits under Medicaid should be expanded. A survey of state Medicaid programs has shown that although home services must be provided by all state Medicaid programs, many states impose restrictions on the amount, duration, and scope of home healthcare visits. In addition, several optional services exist that states may choose to provide, including medical rehabilitation services, adult day care, transportation, and personal care. Twenty-four states provide coverage of personal care services, and 31 provide medical rehabilitation services. Respite care, which would permit families to take a break from caregiving, is not an available service under the regular Medicaid program.

  More than 46 percent of Medicaid's expenditures in 1986 were spent on nursing home care.[4] This reflects the strong institutional bias in the program. The reluctance to expand home health benefits stems from the concern that the availability of benefits will open the floodgates to increased use and higher expenditures. Thus, a need exists to ensure that the services are used in a cost-effective way. The federal government and the states may be less reluctant to expand benefits if some entity or healthcare system assumes some financial risk for providing such services.
- *Provide Care Management*. In the context of a continuum of care, Medicaid expansion should include the component of care management to meet the needs of the poor elderly. A process for assessing the short and long term health and social services needed by Medicaid-eligible elderly is currently lacking. In addition, many states limit home nursing care and home health aide benefits to once or twice a week, although the severely impaired elderly may require daily assistance. The duration of these and other benefits could also be expanded.
- *Increase Medicaid Reimbursement*. The level of Medicaid reimbursement for all providers, especially for nursing homes, should be increased. The increase in reimbursement level should be substantial enough to ensure quality of care. States tend to reimburse facilities at the level necessary for facilities to meet minimum standards for state licensure. With few exceptions, Catholic sponsors and local boards have determined that the level of reimbursement is insufficient to provide the quality of care and personal dignity that their mission calls them to provide. Most Catholic-sponsored facilities subsidize 10 to 40 percent of the cost of care for a resident receiving Medicaid funding. State Medicaid

reimbursement should be increased so that residents directly benefit from this increase. Priority should be given to paying more just wages to the givers of care and, in particular, nursing staffs; improved reimbursement should be structured to pass through nursing salaries. Incentive reimbursement also should be paid for improving the quality of resident life.

Supplemental Security Income

SSI entitles poor elderly age 65 and over to cash assistance. It is a federally administered program that provides this assistance to persons who are aged, blind, or disabled. SSI, although small—less than 1 percent of the federal budget was targeted on the SSI-eligible elderly in fiscal year 1987, or $2.2 billion—is not only important as a welfare program, but also serves as a vehicle for Medicaid enrollment.[5]

The SSI program was established by the 1972 amendments to the Social Security Act under Title XVI and is administered by the Social Security Administration. SSI replaced the former federal grants to the states for old age assistance and aid to blind and permanently disabled persons.

Whereas Social Security benefits are now received by almost all elderly, SSI is received by relatively few. Some elderly receive benefits from both Social Security and SSI.

Strengths and Weaknesses

Recent progress in reducing poverty among the elderly population sometimes obscures the fact that a substantial number of the elderly remain poor. Three and one-half million elderly persons, about 13 percent of all persons aged 65 and older, had incomes below the poverty line in 1985. Poverty is relatively common in elderly female-headed families: it was 23 percent in 1985. The rate for elderly blacks was 31 percent. Poverty, however, is relatively uncommon for elderly married couples, about 6 percent in 1985.[6] Thus, the overall poverty rate for the elderly masks the striking income disparities within the elderly population.

The federal benefit guarantee, however, falls short of the poverty line of $104.75 per week for an elderly person. For example, the federal SSI benefit for single persons (the most common living circumstance for the elderly poor) is equal to 76 percent of the aged poverty line. As its name indicates, the program was designed to supplement other income for retired and disabled persons. Since the concept of a minimum Social Security benefit was eliminated in 1981, SSI is the only program that guarantees a basic level of cash income support for the elderly and disabled poor. About half of the states supplement the federal benefit, but in most cases the supplement is modest. The combined federal and state benefits meet the aged poverty line in only four states.

Task Force Recommendations

- *Increase the SSI Benefit.* The federal SSI benefit level should be increased to the aged poverty line. Eventually 1.2 million more persons would be added to the SSI caseload. Federal costs would increase by $5.1 billion. The poverty rate would drop to 8 percent if the federal guarantee were set at the aged poverty line. This represents about a 38 percent reduction in the prevalence of elderly poverty.
- *Supplement the SSI Benefit.* The SSI benefit rate should be increased for those recipients over age 75. After that age, the likelihood of increased frailty associated with poor health and disability can cause grave financial burdens, thereby consuming a greater portion of available income.
- *Expand Eligibility.* The age of eligibility should be lowered to age 62. Providing eligibility to persons aged 62 to 64 would increase the SSI caseload by 228,000 persons, many of whom are poor elderly widows.
- *Increase Participation.* Approximately 50 percent of the aged who are eligible for benefits actually participate in the program. In general, persons with the greatest need have the highest participation rates. Concerted efforts could be made to increase entitlement among those who are eligible. States should also be required to offer Medicaid benefits to persons eligible for but not participating in SSI.
- *Relax the Asset Test.* Currently, elderly persons are eligible for SSI if they meet an asset test, which was fixed at $1,500 for an individual and $2,250 for a couple when the federal program was designed in 1974. Recent changes have raised the limits to $2,000 for a single person and $3,000 for a couple effective in 1989. These limits are a concern for the aged poor. Those who set aside savings for their retirement are penalized relative to those having only retirement savings in the form of Social Security. The asset limits could be raised to increase eligibility for SSI.
- *Change the Provisions Regarding Recipients Living with Relatives.* Currently, SSI benefits are reduced by one-third for recipients who reside with a relative. This policy should be rescinded since recipients should not suffer discrimination on the basis of where they choose to reside.

Older Americans Act

Two major federal funding sources exist for social services for the elderly: the Older Americans Act, administered by the Administration on Aging, and the Social Services Block Grant Act, administered through the Office of Human Development of the Department of Health and Human

Services (HHS). As another example of the incremental approach, federal funds for these programs are provided to state agencies on a population-based formula. States administer the programs through local agencies.

The purpose of the Older Americans Act is to establish a comprehensive system of community-based services for the elderly. The goal of the legislation is to enable the elderly to live in their own homes with the greatest degree of independence possible. Since the funds are to be used to make continued home living possible, a variety of critical supportive services are provided. Local area agencies on aging are given considerable latitude in deciding how the money is spent. As such, they are well positioned to play an important part in the continuum of care, notably in community-based social services.

In fiscal year 1985, Congress appropriated $669 million for Older Americans Act programs, most of which went to the direct provision of support services, congregate housing, and home-delivered meals. The act prohibits the use of a means test for its programs, but providers must target their efforts on those persons age 60 or older in greatest social and economic need.

The Social Services Block Grant was funded at a level of $2.7 billion in fiscal year 1984. Among the types of services available to qualified elderly persons in most states are home-based services, information and referral, counseling, adult day care, and residential care and treatment.

Another federally funded service program for the elderly is the Older America Volunteer Program administered by the ACTION agency. The Senior Community Service Block Grant administered in HHS also provides some services to the elderly as part of a program serving low-income persons of all ages.

The federal role in the provision of social services is modest compared to its contribution to the income and health needs of the elderly. Estimates indicate that federal social services comprise about 1 percent of federal outlays targeted on the elderly. Local and state governments and the private sector, including family, friends, neighbors, and philanthropic organizations, provide the bulk of social services for the elderly.

Strengths and Weaknesses

The major weakness of these Older Americans Act initiatives is their limited scope. For example, the Social Services Block Grant funding for community care is minimal compared to funding for institutional care. Another weakness is that these programs are subject to local political pressures on funding.

One of the most useful attributes of the Older Americans Act is that few restrictions exist on how local agencies on aging can expend their resources. In fact, some state agencies have served as catalysts to more effectively provide social and health services funded through other programs.

Task Force Recommendation

- *Increase Federal Funding of Social Services for the Elderly.* Increase funding of both Older Americans Act programs and Social Services Block Grants to enable current services to be expanded and new services to be developed. The funding increase would allow additional numbers of elderly to be served.

Housing

Housing assistance for the elderly is available through public programs that include subsidized public housing, rental assistance programs, elderly housing loans, and Farmers Home Administration rental assistance. These programs account for about 2 percent of federal outlays targeted on the elderly.

The public housing program and the Section 8 program are designed to increase the supply of affordable housing for low-income individuals eligible for federal rental assistance. In 1984, almost one half of the 2.5 million public housing units constructed in the United States through these two programs were occupied by elderly persons. In addition, more than 400,000 newly constructed subsidized units were occupied by the elderly.

The Section 202 loan program, traditionally thought of as the elderly housing program, is designed specifically to construct low-income rental housing for elderly and nonelderly handicapped persons. The program is mandated to have all sponsors classified as private, not-for-profit organizations. More than one-half of the program sponsors have been religious institutions. Approximately 155,000 units constructed under the Section 202 direct loan program were occupied by elderly persons in 1984, which represents less than 10 percent of federally assisted units for the elderly. As the National Housing Task Force concluded in its report, an increasing number of frail elderly who are poor and can no longer live independently cannot find appropriate housing.

In recent years, total new commitments for Section 8 housing fell from 206,000 units in 1980 to 100,000 units for 1984.[7] The Congressional Budget Office reports total housing assistance outlays for all persons were reduced by $1.8 billion for 1982 to 1985 compared to previous policy, the result of reduced new commitments. Because housing commitments are long term, the effects of the decreased outlays will continue far into the future. Moreover, under new eligibility rules, about one fifth of those elderly households residing in assisted housing will be ineligible.

The provision increasing rents to 30 percent of countable income will make one in nine participating elderly households ineligible. All changes combine to eliminate eligibility for about one fourth of participating elderly households.

Task Force Recommendations

- *Relax Existing Eligibility Criteria for the Elderly.* The eligibility criteria for participating in housing assistance should be relaxed to allow more elderly households to qualify.
- *Increase Funding.* Additional funding should be allocated to increase the available supply of rental housing for the elderly.
- *Increase Availability of Congregate Housing.* With the help of the Administration on Aging, congregate housing is spreading to rural areas, where prevalence of elderly poverty is the greatest and where 60 percent of the nation's substandard housing is located. Additional funding of congregate housing assistance is required to provide this needed link in the continuum of care spectrum.

The Veterans Administration

The Veterans Administration (VA) healthcare system was designed primarily to assist veterans with service-connected injuries or low incomes, but it also serves those with illnesses and injuries unrelated to their service and those with middle-to-upper incomes. Many analysts believe the VA system is a model of comprehensive medical and social services for veterans.

The VA provides a range of long term care services, including nursing home care, outpatient visits, placement in special housing, personal care, adult day care services, and hospice care. Through the VA's geriatric evaluation units at its hospitals, medical and social problems of older veterans are identified and assessed. The purpose of this approach is to reduce rehospitalization and nursing home placement. Social workers attempt to find alternative forms of care that are more appropriate to the patient's needs.

Strengths and Weaknesses

The VA healthcare system targets the older veteran and has designed a comprehensive set of services for their needs. One of its strengths is its aim to reduce rehospitalization and nursing home placement through specialized geriatric evaluation units.

The VA's greatest weakness is that, as a federal program, it will compete with other programs for financial support. As a result, this system, which will have the responsibility for taking care of ever-greater numbers of people, may be underfunded.

The Future: Long Term Care Insurance

The financing and delivery of long term care for the elderly is very complex. At least four major federal programs cover nursing care facilities and home and community-based services: Medicaid, Medicare, Social Service Block Grants, and the Older Americans Act. But gaps still exist; for example, Medigap policies, which supplement Medicare, do not cover long term care.

Medicaid is the largest federal program for long term care. Once eligible for Medicaid, payment for care will be assumed by the government. Public benefits are reduced dollar for dollar for any out-of-pocket financial contributions made by the patient or family. In some instances, Medicaid may only cover impaired elderly admitted to institutions, but not those who could remain at home and wish to do so.

Assessment of Public and Private Options

Private Insurance. Private insurance policies for long term care have existed for some time but cover only 150,000 individuals and contribute less than 1 percent to the total cost of long term care for the elderly. The low rate of coverage results from its relatively high cost and from the general erroneous perception that either Medicare or Medicaid will automatically pay for long term care. However, more employers such as American Express and the states of Alaska, Maryland, and Ohio are sponsoring long term care group coverage for their employees.[8] A need exists for insurance companies, consumer groups, provider groups, and organizations representing older persons to make consumers aware of the lack of long term care coverage by Medicare and private insurance. Among the recommendations to facilitate the purchase of long term care insurance made by the congressionally established Task Force on Long Term Care was the suggestion that individuals should be allowed to make tax-free transfers from retirement funds. This measure, however, would be applicable only to those elderly persons with sufficient resources to purchase long term care insurance. Also, tax incentives would be offered to employers as an inducement to include long term care coverage in their employee health plans.

Payments to Family Members. A few states authorize the use of Medicaid funds to pay family members to care for their elderly relatives; more should do so in the future. Medicaid allows family members to be reimbursed only through special provisions of the Home and Community-Based Care program. Proponents argue that payment enhances family care, whereas critics charge that the public is paying for services that would have been provided free of charge anyway. As part of its pension program, the VA provides a "constant attendance allowance" to more than 220,000 veterans and/or their dependents who require the ongoing assistance of another person.

Medical Individual Retirement Accounts. The concept of medical individual retirement accounts (IRAs), similar to retirement IRAs, is another option to finance long term care. A medical IRA could be established to finance individual expenses for chronic care. They would be optional and would be sheltered from certain taxes. Their applicability is limited to those with sufficient resources. Also, some tax drain would amount to a subsidy to those individuals who can afford or who choose to save in this way. On the other hand, encouraging persons to save during their working years may obviate the necessity for government to expend resources in the future for those who have assumed individual responsibility for their retirement years.

Tax Incentives. Federal income taxes provide limited subsidies to families who purchase dependent care for their elderly members living at home. Under the Economic Recovery Act of 1981, the federal tax structure was expanded to allow a tax credit for noninstitutional care for a disabled spouse or other dependent. Previously, the tax credits only applied to the care of children under age 15. Certain qualifications must be met to receive the credit: care must be provided outside the home; the disabled person must spend at least 8 hours per day in the taxpayer's home, and all taxpayers must be gainfully employed. Arizona, Idaho, Oregon, and Iowa have similar tax provisions in their state income tax laws for the care of the dependent elderly.

Social Health Maintenance Organization. A social health maintenance organization (SHMO) is a managed system of health and long term care services. A single provider entity assumes responsibility for a full range of acute inpatient, ambulatory, rehabilitative, extended care, home health, and personal care services. Nursing home benefits are limited to three to six months. In the early 1980s, the Health Care Financing Administration and private foundations sponsored a project to develop the SHMO concept. The projects, which began enrollment in March 1985, are phasing in enrollment and will gradually absorb more risk over three and one-half years. The success of the SHMO model, however, is still being evaluated.

Home and Community-Based Medicaid Waivers. Home and community-based Medicaid waivers cover a broad range of services designed to maintain an impaired elderly person in a noninstitutional setting who would otherwise reside in Medicaid-financed institutions. The services are not necessarily medical, and many include assistance from housekeepers, home health aides, transportation services, adult day care, and respite care. The program became an option for state Medicaid agencies in October 1983. States, however, must obtain waivers to exempt them from current Medicaid restrictions. The purpose is to ensure appropriate placement in nursing care facilities or other community-based services. In the past, Medicaid could not pay for housekeeper services because they were not medically oriented services. Moreover, many impaired elderly were not eligible for Medicaid until after they were admitted to an institution. Medicaid waiver projects such as those conducted in Oregon have not resolved all the existing fragmentation, but each seems to make some progress toward a more coherent system. Although the full impact is not yet known and may vary from state to state, the expected savings from the program have yet to be demonstrated.

Financing Options

A client-focused, coordinated continuum of care for the frail elderly will require not only integration of the various services, but also a method of financing that will increase available monetary resources. The vision of quality long term care will require a sizable financial investment. The following are options to be considered in paying for that vision.

Taxing Social Security Benefits. In 1983, Congress passed a package of amendments to the Social Security Act that represented a bipartisan effort to deal with serious near-term and long-range financing problems facing the OASDI program. A key feature of this legislation was the introduction of Social Security benefit taxation. Beginning in 1984, partial taxation of benefits was introduced. One half of Social Security benefits is added to adjusted gross income of single persons with income above $25,000 and couples with income above $32,000 as the threshold to trigger tax liability.

An appealing feature of increasing Social Security benefit taxation is not only that it is closely identified with the population that we wish to assist, but also that revenue generated through the personal income tax system can and should easily be earmarked for the SSI program.

Increasing the Payroll Tax. Another option is to increase the amount of earned income subject to the FICA payroll tax. In 1988, the limit is $45,000. The limit could be increased or the cap eliminated. Since the payroll tax is earmarked for programs that provide benefits to elderly and disabled persons, it is a logical device for financing improvement in the protection against poverty that would be provided to the elderly. In addition, the burden from an increase in the maximum taxable wage would fall on those most able to pay, making the tax a bit less regressive. Many are likely to resist this mechanism, since it will be perceived as onerous to high-wage workers.

Increasing Inheritance Tax. The ceiling on income exempt from inheritance taxes could be frozen at the current $600,000 level. Alternatively, if the estate tax exemption were lowered to $400,000, federal revenues would increase by approximately $9 billion over the 1987-1991 period. In addition, the top marginal tax rate could be kept at its current level of 55 percent and not lowered to 50 percent as is scheduled for 1988. Alternatively, this rate could be raised.

Although increasing inheritance taxes is politically unpopular, one advantage in using the estate tax to finance improvements for the elderly is that the purchasing power of the elderly would be unaffected during their lifetimes.

Taxing Capital Gains. A modest proposal to tax capital gains at death could generate sufficient funds to reduce some elderly poverty.

Increasing Alcohol and Cigarette Tax. Increased taxes on alcohol and cigarettes could serve a dual purpose: curtailing consumption of goods that impose costs to society in the form of higher healthcare expenditures, and raising revenue to pay for the costs incurred.

Conclusion

The growing number of elderly-persons-at-risk have set the foundation for a call to action, to commitment, and to caring for both the whole Church and Catholic healthcare providers. The complex and fluctuating needs of the most frail among us compel the Task Force to share its heightened sense of urgency with all who come in contact with the elderly-at-risk. The Church, in its role as educator, protector, and advocate for all God's people, is summoned to address its resources to the special vulnerability of the frail elderly. One of the Church's great strengths in recognizing this demographic phenomenon is its network of medical facilities and social agencies. On this already impressive array of building blocks, the framework for addressing the future of long term care for the frail elderly can be built.

Providers of Catholic healthcare have an equally demanding role to play in ensuring that the elderly-at-risk receive the most humane and appropriate response to their need for services. While no single facility or agency is ideally suited to coordinate the continuum, the potential for Catholic healthcare providers to demonstrate leadership within the community and to become an active participant in the continuum of care is uniquely opportune in this moment of history. The ever-increasing numbers of elderly are forcing Catholic healthcare providers to rethink basic strategy in coping not only with the elderly's health and social needs, but with their access to both.

The successful continuum of care, with its client focus, its array of appropriate services, and its integrating coordination, ensures that the values and goals articulated in Chapter 2 find their fullest expression in healthcare for the elderly-at-risk. As part of the vision, the continuum of care builds on the informal supports already in place and substitutes for them when they are absent. Access to the continuum for the frail elderly person is negotiated by the care management component and is financially and geographically available to the client. As the functional states of the elderly person change, the continuum responds by making a reassessment and offering newly appropriate services. Clients are constantly moving about within the continuum, with each changing level of need being met. The dignity and autonomy of the frail person are at the very core of the truly successful continuum.

Jesus sought out the hungry, the sick, and the elderly and ministered to them. The Task Force believes that the elderly-at-risk remain a hidden reality about to burst forth on our consciousness. This report attempts to respond to that need by proposing a new vision of long term care for the frail elderly.

NOTES

1. "1988 Annual Report of the Board of Trustees of the Federal Hospital Insurance Trust Fund," Washington, DC, U.S. Department of Health and Human Services, May 1988.
2. *Social Security Bulletin Annual Statistical Supplement 1987,* Washington, DC, U.S. Department of Health and Human Services.
3. HCFA (1986). HCFA program statistics. *Health Care Financing Review* 4: 127-132.
4. Alice M. Rivlin and Joshua M. Wiener, *Caring for the Disabled Elderly: Who Will Pay?* Washington, DC, The Brookings Institution, 1988.
5. Rosalie A. Kane and Robert L. Kane, *Long Term Care: Principles, Programs, and Policies,* New York, Springer Publishing Co., 1987, p. 71.
6. "Old, Alone and Poor: A Plan for Reducing Poverty Among Elderly People Living Alone," Baltimore, The Commonwealth Fund Commission on Elderly People Living Alone, 1987.
7. "A Decent Place To Live," The Report of the National Housing Task Force, Washington, DC, March 1988.
8. "Nursing Home Care as a Working Benefit," *The Wall Street Journal,* June 30, 1988.

Glossary

When a term appears in **boldface** within a definition, a separate definition of it will be found elsewhere in the glossary.

A

activities of daily living (instrumental and basic) physical functions that an independent person performs each day. Instrumental activities of daily living include housekeeping, transportation, food preparation, grocery shopping, etc. Basic activities of daily living include **personal care services** such as bathing, eating, grooming, walking, dressing, and toilet use.

acute care treatment provided, either on an inpatient or **outpatient** basis, for **acute**, as opposed to **chronic disease**. Acute illness is usually of short duration, and the patient usually returns to his/her previous condition. An episode of a chronic illness (e.g., diabetic coma in a patient with diabetes) is often treated as an acute illness. An acute care (or short stay) facility is one where the average length of stay is less than 30 days.

acute disease an **illness** characterized by a single episode of fairly short duration, from which the patient returns to his/her normal or previous state and level of activity. While acute disease is frequently distinguished from **chronic disease** there is no standard definition or distinction. An acute episode of a chronic illness (e.g., leukemia, or an episode of diabetic coma in a patient with diabetes) is often treated as an acute illness.

adult day care service service provided for part of a day and in a congregate setting to individuals who can benefit from care but do not require institutionalization. This may include meals, **personal care services**, and recreational and educational activities. See also **adult day health service**.

adult day health service program of **health** and supporting services provided under auspices of a healthcare facility or freestanding adult day healthcare center for adults who do not require 24-hour care and, yet, due to social, physical and/or mental impairments, are not capable of full-time independent living. Supervised day health programs are designed to provide the maximum support to an elderly person who, because of mobility and/or chronic conditions, would be at great risk were it not for the program. Participants receive a complete screening to assess their needs with a defined plan of daily activities and therapies. Specific conditions of participation apply in states which license such programs. Such rules often govern staffing, physical plant, transfer requirements, and programs.

adult foster care service offered in the private home of an individual or family who offers board and shelter (meals, housekeeping, minimal surveillance, and **personal care**) to one or more unrelated ("foster") adults.

adult night care service service provided for part of a night and in a congregate setting for individuals requiring supervision but not institutionalization. This service may be used as **respite** for the patient's family.

advance directives any general or specific statement made by someone who *anticipates* a time in the future when he/she may no longer be competent to make decisions about his/her healthcare; it is intended to *direct* healthcare professionals, family, and friends who will be making those decisions on his/her behalf.

alcoholism a **chronic disease** manifested by habitual drinking of alcoholic beverages in excess of dietary needs, social uses, and norms of the community, and to the extent that it interferes with the drinker's **health**, social, or economic functioning. It is difficult to define alcoholism precisely, either in theory or practice. Excessive drinking may or may not interfere with a person's functioning; and if it does, it may or may not be accompanied by physical signs of **drug dependence**. Alcohol and **substance abuse** may require either long-term or short-term treatment programs, or a combination of both, and often requires admission to a hospital or **rehabilitation** facility.

assessment gathering of data to identify the client's assets and the areas in which assistance or supportive services are needed. The assessment tool used to collect the data should address physical, cognitive, functional, environmental, social, and spiritual needs.

assessment unit a formal, structured service unit organized to conduct multidisciplinary assessment of a person's status, problems, needs, and abilities. The assessment is conducted by professionals from several disciplines such as medicine, nursing, and social work. A service program is designed to meet the person's needs as identified through the assessment. The assessment unit may be freestanding or associated with a program or facility such as a hospital, **nursing home**, or day health program.

assisted living a service in which elderly or impaired persons receive assistance for a variety of daily chores (e.g., shopping, meals, housekeeping, personal needs).

B

boarding home an organized or informal facility that provides room and board and sometimes **supportive care**. Since medical supervision, social activities, and counseling are not normally included, boarding homes in most states are not subject to any licensure requirements.

C

care (case) management (also known as **service management**) a comprehensive and continuous process of developing, coordinating, and sustaining multiple services for a client. On the basis of an initial **assessment** of the person's needs, the assigned care manager assumes responsibility for providing a service plan that considers all available service solutions and assures both that the client is actually referred to service and that progress is examined at regular intervals. See also **discharge planning.**

catastrophic health insurance insurance that provides protection against the high cost of treating severe or lengthy **illnesses** or **disabilities**. Such insurance policies generally cover all or a specified percentage of medical expenses above an amount which is the responsibility of the insured person or of another insurance policy up to a maximum limit of liability. Coverage typically begins after the insured has incurred medical expenses equal to a deductible amount (e.g., $5,000 within a 12-month period), or a specified percentage of one's income (e.g., 15 percent), or has been in a medical institution for a specified period (e.g., 60 days). Individuals (or another insurance policy, if the person is so covered) are liable for all costs up to the specified limits. While there is generally no maximum amount of coverage under these plans, many include some coinsurance.

chemical dependence a synonym for **drug dependence**. See also **substance abuse**.

chore services: see **homemaker service.**

chronic care hospital a facility that provides care for patients who require higher levels of care than that provided by **skilled nursing facilities**, facilities including almost daily care or observation by a **physician**, preferably one who specializes in **rehabilitation** medicine. Also known as a **chronic disease** hospital or **long term care** hospital.

chronic disease an **illness** which has one or more of the following characteristics: it is permanent; leaves residual **disability**; is caused by irreversible pathological alteration; requires special training of the patient for **rehabilitation**; or may be expected to require a long period of supervision, observation, or care. See also **acute disease, long term care**.

congregate care home: see **congregate housing.**

congregate housing a facility that provides a sheltered living environment for residents, possibly including such services as housekeeping, meals, social activities, protective oversight, assistance with **personal care** activities, and intervention in a crisis situation. The scope of services to residents ranges from very limited personal services in an independent living environment to a full-service supportive living environment.

congregate meal service food service provided to an elderly population in such congregate settings as **senior citizen centers** and **congregate housing**.

community mental health center an entity which provides comprehensive **mental health services**, principally on an outpatient basis and primarily to individuals residing or employed in a defined service area. The term is defined in the Community Mental Health Centers Act (section 201) which specifies the services to be provided and the requirements for the governance, organization, and operation of the centers.

conservator a guardian; protector; preserver. A person or corporation appointed by a court to provide care for a minor or a disabled person and have custody of his/her estate.

continuing care retirement community (CCRC) an organization established to provide **housing** and services, including healthcare to people of retirement age. At a minimum, the community meets each of the following criteria: 1) campus consists of independent living units; it may also contain healthcare facilities such as **congregate housing**, **personal care**, and **intermediate** or **skilled nursing**; 2) community offers a contract that lasts for more than one year and guarantees shelter and various healthcare services; 3) fees for healthcare services are less than the full cost of such services and have been partly prepaid by the resident.

continuum of care the availability of a coordinated, integrated, array of effective **long term care** services with an explicit client focus. The range of services is comprehensive and covers the spectrum from social-intensive, community-based, primarily outpatient care to health-intensive, institution-based, primarily inpatient care. The continuum's primary focus is on the needs and preferences of those being served. The integrating elements of planning, care management, a management information system, financing, and administrative structure form the bridge between clients and services, and distinguish a true continuum from other sets of services simply having an information and referral system.

contract service specialized service, such as **physical therapy** or nutrition, provided for the clientele or agency through a contractual agreement. Such services as computer time or laundry may also be provided by contract between one agency and another.

D

day care: see **adult day care**, **adult day health service**.

day hospital a facility designed to provide **acute care** services (e.g., minor surgery, chemotherapy, diagnosis, and treatment) that do not require an overnight stay. While a day hospital has certain characteristics in common with an acute care hospital, it is more like an **outpatient care facility**, but with medical resources sufficient to provide certain services normally available only in a hospital. Day hospitals provide comprehensive **assessment**, **rehabilitation**, and specific therapy, and can be specialized for special groups such as geriatric or psychiatric clients.

diagnosis related group (DRGs) classification system which uses diagnostic information to establish hospital payments under Medicare. This system groups patient needs into 467 categories, based upon the coding system of the *International Classification of Diseases*, 9th Revision—Clinical Modification (ICD-9-CM).

disability any curtailment of an individual's physical, mental, or social activity, as compared with persons of similar age, sex, and occupation. Disability frequently refers to any limitation of a person's usual or major activities, especially those connected with one's occupation. Disability is of varying types (functional, vocational, learning), degrees (partial, total), and durations (temporary, permanent), and may require **long term care** or **rehabilitation**. Disability benefits are often available only for specific disabilities, such as total and permanent (the requirement for Social Security and **Medicare**).

discharge planning portion of patient care planning that concentrates on a patient's readiness for discharge or transfer to another level of care and the activities needed to arrange community services following discharge.

disease a failure of the adaptive mechanism of an organism to counteract adequately, normally, or appropriately the stimuli and stresses to which it is subject, resulting in a disturbance in the function or structure of some part of the organism. This definition emphasizes that disease has many factors and may be prevented or treated by changing the factors. In fact, disease is a very elusive concept to define, being determined largely by social acceptance. Thus, criminal behavior, **alcoholism**, and **drug dependence** tend now to be seen as diseases, whereas in the past they were considered to be moral or legal problems. See also **acute disease**, **chronic disease**, and **illness**.

domiciliary care home: see **congregate housing.**

drug abuse persistent or sporadic drug use inconsistent with or unrelated to acceptable medical or cultural practice. The definition of drug abuse is imprecise, sometimes also designating excessive use of a drug, unnecessary use (thus including recreational use), illegal use, and **drug dependence**. See also **alcoholism, substance abuse**.

drug dependence a psychic, and sometimes also physical, condition resulting from the interaction between a person and a drug, characterized by behavioral and other responses that always include a compulsion to take the drug on a regular basis in order to experience its psychic effects, and sometimes to avoid the discomfort and other physical effects of its withdrawal or absence. The user may or may not be able to tolerate the drug, and may be dependent on more than one drug. The characteristics of drug dependence vary with the substance involved, and this must be made clear in each case: e.g., drug dependence of a narcotic type, cannabis type, barbiturate or amphetamine type, etc.

Drug dependence may or may not be severe, illegal, or harmful to the dependent individual (e.g., a terminally ill patient under **hospice** treatment) or to society. See also **drug abuse**, **alcoholism**.

durable medical equipment: see **medical equipment and supplies, home health care.**

durable power of attorney a power of attorney which continues in existence for the life of the grantor after the incompetency of the grantor has been established (whether adjudged or not); except that, if a guardian or conservator is appointed, the appointing court has the discretion to terminate the durable power of attorney. The concept of the durable power of attorney has been adopted by statute in most states but has not been frequently used in treatment decisions.

E

extended care in **Medicare**, services provided in a **skilled nursing facility**: specifically, **nursing care** requiring a professional registered nurse; room and board; **physical**, **occupational**, or **speech therapy**; medical social services; medication, supplies, and equipment ordinarily used in caring for skilled nursing facility patients; certain **physician** services; and other services necessary to patients' **health**.

extended care facility previously used in **Medicare** to designate a **skilled nursing facility (SNF)** which qualified for participation in Medicare. In 1972, the law was amended to use the more generic term "skilled nursing facility" for both Medicare and **Medicaid.** Medicare coverage is limited to 100* days of post-hospital **extended care** services during any spell of **illness,** when the services are related to the cause of the hospital stay. These conditions do not apply to SNF benefits under Medicaid. Thus, the continued use of the term "extended care facility benefits" is a convenient way of referring to the benefit limitations on SNF care under Medicare.

*(150 days effective Jan. 1, 1989)

F

family and patient education programs programs of **health education** or **health promotion** designed to foster good **health**, prevent **illness**, and encourage more healthful habits. See also **health promotion**.

financial counseling a social service for elderly and other persons aimed at maximizing needed income and the efficient use of financial resources.

formal caregiver persons trained to provide direct care service (i.e., home health aide) for a fee. (Informal caregiver is a family member, friend, or volunteer that has not received formal education to provide care and does not receive a fee for services provided.)

foster care: see **adult foster care.**

friendly visiting personal, regularly scheduled visitation of homebound or socially isolated individuals for the purpose of assuring continuing contact with the community.

functional assessment a formalized process for determining the nature of a person's ability to perform certain functions such as personal care, household tasks, and the like, to identify needed services, or to monitor a person's progress. Functional assessment may also include a **physical assessment** which focuses on a person's physical status.

functional maintenance services: see **rehabilitation.**

G

geriatrics medical treatment of age-associated disease.

geriatric clinic an **outpatient care facility** which provides services to the elderly, usually **geriatric medical services**, but sometimes also nonmedical, social, and counseling services.

geriatric day rehabilitation hospital: see **day hospital.**

geriatric medical services services of medical nature (such as dental, podiatry, nursing) for elderly persons, as distinguished from **social work** services and **personal care** (or personal **health**) services. May be provided in an inpatient or clinic setting.

geriatrician a **physician** who specializes in providing medical care especially to older adults.The usual background of a geriatrician includes formal medical education, specializaton in internal medicine or family practice, and further special training in geriatric medicine, preparing him/her for work with a **team** of professionals in order to maximize the functional abilities of the older adult.

geriatric nurse practitioner (GNP) a **registered nurse** educationally prepared to assume an expanding role in providing primary healthcare to older persons and their families; one who possesses extensive knowledge of **physical assessment** and can manage stable **chronic** and minor **acute diseases** or conditions afflicting older persons; and who collaborates with other health professionals to provide optimal care to older persons. GNPs are certified for expanded practice within a state.

geriatric nurse clinical specialist a **registered nurse**, who, through study and supervised practice at the graduate level (master's or doctorate), has become expert in a selected clinical area of nursing service for elderly patients, and who is eligible for specialty certification through nursing's professional society.

gerontology the scientific study of the social and biological process of aging and of the problems (physical, spiritual, and social) of aged people. See also **geriatrics**.

geropsychiatrist or psychogeriatrician a **physician** who specializes in providing psychiatric care to older adults. The usual background of a geropsychiatrist includes formal medical education, specialization in psychiatry, and further special training in geriatric psychiatry, preparing him/her for work with a **team** of professionals in order to maximize the functional abilities of the older adult.

group home an organizationally sponsored living arrangement shared by several older adults. Tenants or residents are jointly responsible for food preparation, housekeeping, and recreation. Group homes usually do not need a license and do not provide healthcare or **personal care services**.

guarantor one who undertakes collaterally to answer for the payment of another's debt or the performance of another's duty, liability, or obligation; typically, a guarantor's promise is not enforceable until it can be shown to some legal standard that the other person has failed to pay the debt or perform the duty or obligation. In general, a guarantor agrees to pay on a contracted debt upon the principal's failure or inability to pay.

guardian in a context relating to property rights or obligations, the guardian is the conservator of the estate. When used in a context relating to rights and obligations other than property or obligations, it means **guardian of the person.**

guardian of the person the one appointed by a court to have custody of and care for a minor or incapacitated person.

guardian ad litem one appointed by a court, in which particular litigation is pending, to represent a minor, an incapacitated person, a disabled person, or an unborn person in that particular proceeding or as otherwise specified by the law of the jurisdiction.

H

health state of complete physical, mental, spiritual, and social well-being, and not merely the absence of **disease** and infirmity.

health education information and instruction provided in many settings by various health workers (including professional health educators) on such topics as accident prevention, diet, diagnosis of physical illness, psychological aid, self-administration of medication, and improvements in healthful living standards. The purpose of health education is to modify behavior and encourage a more healthful lifestyle. See also **health promotion.**

health insurance insurance against loss resulting from **acute** or **chronic disease,** bodily injury, or other conditions requiring **acute care** or chronic care. Government-sponsored health insurance programs include **Medicare, Medicaid,** CHAMPUS, and CHAMPVA; Blue Cross, Blue Shield, and commercial insurance plans are those offered by private-sector, and often for-profit, insurance companies. See also **catastrophic health insurance, health maintenance organization.**

health maintenance organization (HMO) a health delivery system that agrees to provide or otherwise ensure the delivery of certain basic or supplemental health services to a voluntarily enrolled group of subscribers, in return for a predetermined fixed periodic payment. Unlike insured fee-for-service, where the insurance carrier (rather than the provider) is at risk, an HMO is both the provider of services and the party at risk for any financial losses. Because of this, HMOs and **preferred provider arrangements** (sometimes call **managed care plans**) must "manage" (i.e., exercise strict control over) the use and cost of services, and rarely if ever cover **nursing home** care. Between 1981 and 1985, HMO enrollment grew from 10.3 million to 21.1 million, while the number of HMOs rose from 243 to 480.

At the start of 1986, close to 1 million **Medicare** beneficiaries and about one-half million **Medicaid** beneficiaries were enrolled in HMOs.

health promotion any of numerous programs aimed at fostering good **health** and preventing **illness;** e.g., **wellness programs,** exercise classes, **family and patient education programs,** nutrition consultation, meal programs, and volunteer programs. See also **health education, preventive medicine.**

health protection or **prevention** services aimed at guarding or defending the person from injury such as **illness,** disturbances and relationships, or social disruption.

home-delivered meal service a service which delivers ready-to-eat meals to individuals at home; sometimes known by such names as **Meals on Wheels,** Mobile Meals, etc.

home healthcare care provided to individuals and families in their place of residence, for the purpose of promoting, maintaining, or restoring **health,** or of maximizing the level of independence, while minimizing the effects of **disability** and **illness,** including terminal illness. Service needs are determined by a multidisciplinary **team** or a single health professional, and are planned, coordinated, and delivered by providers organized to do so through the use of employed staff, contractual arrangements, or a combination of the two. Services may include any of the following components: medical, dental, pharmacy, or laboratory, as well as other **medical equipment and supplies; home infusion therapies; homemaker service; hospice; nursing care;** nutrition, **physician** services, **social work** and counseling; **speech, physical, occupational, and rehabilitation therapy,** and **transportation services.**

Some home healthcare agencies are **Medicare**-certified. Medicare Part B (Supplemental Medical Insurance) will pay 80 percent of reasonable costs for covered **physician** services and 100 percent of reasonable charges for home health agency visits, subject to certain cost limits.

home infusion therapy any form of intravenous therapy administered as part of **home healthcare.**

home repair service a service that provides repairs and modifications to a person's living quarters, with the objective of maintaining or increasing the person's ability to perform activities of daily living, or of eliminating unsafe conditions. The service includes: assessing the adequacy of the person's residence in relation to individual needs; recommending needed repairs and structural adaptations; and carrying out such tasks as adding ramps, improving doorways, making minor floor and roof repairs, repairing windows, coolers, and heaters, and installing grab bars, safety mats, and screens.

homemaker service nonmedical services such as cleaning, laundry, meal preparation, and shopping, provided to an individual living at home but unable to perform these activities. Also called **chore services,** these programs are distinguished from **personal care services,** in that the latter are directed at the person, while the former are directed at the individual's environment. Personal care and homemaker services may be provided concurrently and by the same health worker or volunteer.

hospice a program that provides palliative and **supportive care** for the terminally ill and support services for their families. The principal hospice services include **home health care,** inpatient care, counseling, education, and bereavement services. The hospice movement began in the 1970s at St. Christopher's Hospice near London. One of the first hospice programs in the United States was begun at the Yale-New Haven Hospital. In October 1983, **Medicare** expanded its hospital **insurance** benefits to include hospice care for terminally ill Medicare beneficiaries.

housing (elderly) living accommodations which are designed to suit the special needs of the elderly and which may include some components of medical and nonmedical service. See also **adult foster care, boarding home, congregate care home, domiciliary care home, geriatric day rehabilitation hospital, group home, hospice, independent housing, respite care, retirement village, senior apartments.**

I

illness although often used as a synonym for **disease,** illness may be said to be present when an individual perceives himself/herself as suffering disease, whereas disease is present when it can be identified by objective external criteria.

independent housing living accommodations for the elderly which do not include any components of medical or nonmedical service, other than usual services for tenants, but where residents are expected to care for their own personal needs. See **housing (elderly).**

informal caregiver those persons not necessarily formally trained to provide direct care or support services to the person in need and at no cost to the person. Usually includes family members, friends, or parish volunteers.

information and referral service a service which provides information regarding the availability and eligibility requirements of direct service programs, and which facilitates initial contact with the needed service provider. This may include making an appointment or simply referring the person to the provider. Many hospitals now have a **physician** referral service by telephone.

insurance: see **health insurance.**

intermediate care facility (ICF) an institution licensed to provide health related care and services to persons who do not require the degree of care or treatment provided by a hospital or **skilled nursing facility,** but who require care or services available only through institutional facilities. Such facilities can take people with some impairments in their instrumental **activities of daily living** but not in their basic activities of daily living. These facilities are also known as supportive **nursing care** facilities, or health related facilities.

L

legal service a service providing legal interpretation and consultation related to the basic needs of food, shelter, and income. This may include legal advice on income maintenance and eligibility for health programs, as well as assistance in estate planning, wills, governorships, consumer affairs, employment pensions, social security, owner-tenant relationships, and other matters.

licensed practical nurse a paraprofessional educated and authorized by law (state) to perform certain nursing skills under the direction of a **registered nurse** or **physician.**

life care community a congregate living program in which a variety of **housing,** health, and recreational services are provided for more than a year, and often for the rest of the resident's life, in return for a contractual fee paid in advance. Also known as life care home.

long term care diagnostic, preventive, therapeutic, rehabilitative, supportive, and maintenance services focused on the needs and preferences of individuals who have **chronic** physical and/or mental impairments in a variety of institutional and noninstitutional health settings, including the home. From this client-focused perspective, long term care is understood as an extended transition from one functional state to another. The objective of long term care is to improve or maintain the health of the patients, to make them as functionally independent as possible, or, in the case of terminally ill patients, to permit them to die peacefully.

long term care in an acute care setting service provided in an acute care facility to patients whose **disability** requires care and supervision of extended duration.

long term care hospital: see **chronic care hospital.**

long term care insurance insurance that provides protection against the costs of **long term care** services. The long term care insurance market is currently in an infancy state and is undergoing rapid change.

M

managed care plan a generic name for prepaid health plans such as **HMOs, PPAs,** and **primary care networks.** Unlike conventional fee-for-service **insurance** plans (where the insurance carrier, and not the provider, is at risk), prepaid plans are both the provider of services and the party at risk for any financial losses. For that reason, they must carefully "manage" (i.e., exercise strict control over) the use and cost of services, and are thus sometimes called managed care plans. The number of managed care plans and their enrollees has risen rapidly in recent years, and includes some under Catholic auspices.

Meals on Wheels: see **home-delivered meal service.**

Medicaid a federally-aided, state-operated and administered program of medical benefits for qualified persons of low income, established as Title XIX of the 1965 Social Security Amendments. The program covers only certain categories of needy persons—the aged, blind, disabled, and members of families with dependent children where one parent is absent, incapacitated, or unemployed. Under broad federal guidelines, each state determines the benefits, eligibility, payment rates, and methods of administering the program. Federal law requires that states participating in the Medicaid program provide at least the following: laboratory and x-ray services; **skilled nursing facility** care and **home healthcare** services for those 21 years of age or older; early and periodic screening, diagnosis, and treatment of persons under 21; family planning services; and rural health clinic services. In 1984 Medicaid provided services to almost 22.7 million persons at a cost of $38.7 billion. Slightly less than half of that total was paid by the states; the balance represents the federal government's share, as determined by a federal medical assistance percentage formula. Unlike **Medicare,** which provides very limited coverage of **long term care** for the elderly, *Medicaid does cover long term care services under certain conditions.*

medical equipment and supplies as included in **home healthcare,** these include: oxygen and oxygen therapy equipment; ostomy products; disposable incontinency products; dialysis equipment and supplies; parenteral/enteral nutrition; hospital-type beds; wheelchairs and walkers; transcutaneous nerve stimulators; ambulatory and toilet aids. Some of these (like wheelchairs and walkers) are called durable medical equipment.

Medicare a federal program of **health insurance** benefits, without regard to the beneficiary's income, for those aged 65 or over, for certain disabled persons, and for certain persons with chronic kidney disease. The program was established as Title XVIII (Health Insurance of the Aged) of the 1965 Social Security Amendments and became effective on July 1, 1966. It consists of two separate but related programs: hospital insurance (Part A) and supplementary medical insurance (Part B). Part A covers all Medicare-eligible persons and requires no premium, but does require a deductible of $520 per benefit period. There is a copayment requirement (per day from Day 61 to Day 90 of a spell of illness, increasing copayment per day for each of 60 lifetime reserve days, and a copayment per day for Days 21 through 100 of **extended care** services in a **skilled nursing facility**). The 1983 Social Security Amendments (PL 98-21) established a prospective payment system for Medicare Part A, based on **diagnosis related groups (DRGs).** Part B is optional, requires a monthly premium, and has a deductible per year. There is a coinsurance requirement of 20 percent of reasonable charges for **physician** services, unless the physician accepts assignment (the rate assigned by Medicare). Medicare Part B is supported by United States Treasury contributions as well as by participants' premiums.

Several changes to Medicare take effect January 1, 1989. First, Part A will cover all inpatient hospitalization costs 365 days/year after the payment of a single annual deductible. Second, the number of covered days in a skilled nursing facility will be extended from 100 days to 150 days. Third, Part A will impose a new supplemental premium that would be based on a beneficiary's federal income tax liability.

mental health service care designed to enhance, sustain, or restore mental health and well-being. When directed by trained mental health professionals, this service may include many different forms of therapeutic intervention such as counseling, group interaction, and drug therapy. Service may be provided at home, in an outpatient setting, or in an institution. Some definitions of mental health service also include recreational and other activity programs.

N

nurse practitioner a **registered nurse** qualified and specially trained to provide **primary care,** including primary healthcare in homes and in ambulatory care facilities. Nurse practitioners generally function under the supervision of a **physician,** but not necessarily in his presence. They are usually salaried rather than paid on a fee-for-service basis. See **geriatric nurse practitioner.**

nurse specialist: see **geriatric nurse clinical specialist.**

nursing assistant (nurse aide) a trained person who performs various **personal care services** and related nonprofessional services necessary in caring for the personal needs and comforts of patients, residents, or clients.

nursing care care intended to assist a person, sick or well, in the performance of those activities contributing to **health** or its recovery (or to a peaceful death), which the individual would perform unaided if he/she had the necessary strength, will, or knowledge. This includes assisting patients in carrying out therapeutic plans initiated by **physicians** and other health professionals, and assisting other members of the medical **team** in performing the nursing function and understanding the health needs of patients. The specific content of nursing care varies in different countries and situations, and it is important to note that, as defined, it is not given only by nurses but also by many other health workers. See also **nurse practitioner.**

nursing homes any one of a wide range of institutions, other than hospitals, that provide various levels of maintenance and personal or **nursing care** to those who are unable to care for themselves and who may have health problems ranging from minimal to very serious. The term includes freestanding institutions, as well as identifiable components of other health facilities, which provide nursing care and related services, **personal care,** and **residential care.** Nursing homes include **skilled nursing facilities, intermediate care facilities,** and **extended care facilities,** but not **boarding homes.**

nursing home follow-up care provided by a **physician** or other healthcare professional for a patient who had been previously treated in an **acute care** setting and is now in a **nursing home.**

O

occupational therapy medically directed treatment of physically and/or mentally **disabled** individuals, by means of constructive activities designed and adapted by a professionally qualified occupational therapist to promote the restoration of useful function.

outpatient care facility a clinic designed to provide a limited or full range of health and medical services to individuals who do not need to be admitted to a hospital or other institution. These services may include **health education** and maintenance, preventive services, diagnosis, treatment, and **rehabilitation, adult day care,** and **acute care** medical services. An outpatient clinic may also function as a **day hospital.**

outpatient care service limited or full spectrum health and medical services (including health screening, **health education** and maintenance, preventive programs, diagnosis, treatment, **rehabilitation, geriatric medical services,** psychosocial counseling, **adult day care,** and **acute care**) for persons living at home or in an institution. Outpatient care services for the elderly may be located in **congregate housing, long term care** facilities, acute care hospitals, or freestanding or satellite clinics. An outpatient clinic may also function as a **day hospital.**

outreach contact initiated by a provider to identify clients in need of services, to provide information about services and benefits, and to encourage the use of appropriate services. Outreach services may identify isolated or underserved individuals or groups, assist them in gaining access to services, and enable providers to assess the need for services. See also **screening clinics,** mobile vans, **discharge planning, care management, information and referral service,** and emergency response system.

P

passive monitoring any of a number of monitoring systems which involve activation of an alarm by the person in need of assistance, or are activated by the absence of activity in or around the household. Passive monitoring systems are known by a variety of brand names.

pastoral care service provided by trained and certified persons, including ordained ministers of religion, to meet the spiritual needs of patients, their families, and the staff of the agency or facility. Some pastoral care professionals receive specialized training and certification in **gerontology** and/or **rehabilitation,** and most work closely with social workers and healthcare professionals.

personal care service nonmedical assistance in such **activities of daily living** as bathing, grooming, dressing, toilet use, eating, and walking, provided to individuals living at home but unable to perform these tasks without assistance. Personal care service differs from **homemaker** or **chore service,** because it directly affects the person rather than his/her environment. Personal care and homemaker services may be provided concurrently and by the same health worker or volunteer.

physical assessment a formalized process for evaluating the nature or extent of a person's physical problems, needs, strengths, and abilities, and for identifying services to meet the needs and/or to maintain or enhance the strengths. See also **assessment unit, functional assessment.**

physical therapy treatment provided by a licensed physical therapist, using physical agents, biomechanical and neurophysiological principles, and assistive devices to relieve pain, restore maximum function, and prevent **disability** following **disease,** injury, or loss of a body part.

physician a professional qualified by education and authorized by law (usually by having obtained a license) to practice medicine. See also **geriatrician.**

physician assistant (PA) a specially trained, licensed (when required), or otherwise credentialed individual who, under the supervision of a **physician,** performs tasks which might otherwise be performed by physicians themselves. These services may be provided in private physician offices, **outpatient care facilities, long term care** facilities, healthcare institutions, or the patient's home. Also known as physician extenders and by other essentially synonymous terms.

power of attorney the grant of authority to another to act in place of the grantor, either for some particular purpose or for the transaction of business in general. See also **durable power of attorney.**

preferred provider arrangement (PPA) sometimes also called a preferred provider organization (PPO), a PPA is a health delivery system in which an organized group of **physicians** and hospitals contracts with employers or insurers to provide comprehensive healthcare services to enrollees on a fee-for-service basis. Unlike an **HMO,** where providers receive a fixed per capita prepayment and are at risk for losses resulting from the use of services ordered or provided, providers in a **PPA** are paid on a fee-for-service basis (sometimes negotiated) and are not at financial risk. Utilization of service, however, is strictly monitored to minimize their cost to the purchaser, and providers who do not conform to utilization standards may be penalized by the PPA. Unlike HMO enrollees, PPA enrollees are not restricted in their choice of a physician, although there is a financial incentive for enrollees to choose a "preferred provider." PPAs are a rapidly growing sector of the health delivery system, and in mid-1985 there were 151 in the United States with more than 1.3 million enrollees. See also **health maintenance organization, managed care plan.**

prepaid health plan a contract between an insurer and one or more subscribers, in which the plan agrees to provide specified medical care services in return for periodic premiums. **Health maintenance organizations (HMOs)** and competitive medical plans (CMPs) are types of prepaid health plans. Beginning in 1985, certain prepaid plans were permitted to enroll **Medicare** beneficiaries in return for their monthly Medicare premium, but were subject to regulatory restrictions. As of January 1987, approximately 145 prepaid health plans had risk contracts with Medicare covering 836,000 senior citizen enrollees. These plans are paid 95 percent of the adjusted average per capita cost per enrollee, adjusted for certain characteristics other than health status.

preventive medicine care aimed at warding off **illnesses** (e.g., immunizations), at early detection of **disease** (e.g., Pap smears), and at inhibiting further deterioration of the body (e.g., exercise, prophylactic surgery, **wellness programs**). Preventive medicine grew out of discoveries in bacteriology, and was at first concerned with specific medical control measures against the agents of infectious disease. With increasing knowledge of nutritional, malignant, and other **chronic diseases,** and on the assumption that most problems are preventable at some stage of their development, the scope of preventive medicine has been extended to include general preventive measures aimed at improving the healthfulness of our environment and our relations with it through such things as avoidance of hazardous substances, modified diet, and family planning. In particular, the promotion of health through altering behavior, especially by **health education** and **wellness programs,** is gaining prominence as a component of preventive care.

primary care care the consumer receives at the point of contact with the healthcare system, as well as continued care of the individual. Such care entails identification, management, and referral of health problems, as well as preventive and promotive health action to maintain the consumer's **health.**

primary caregiver **physicians** and **primary care** specialists involved in family practice, internal medicine, and pediatrics (and/or nurse practitioners).

primary care network a system of providers and facilities responsible for rendering **primary care** services to the enrollees of a **prepaid health plan.** In addition to direct health services, these services may include preadmission screening, referrals to specialists, and the like, and are designed to ensure that care is provided in the most economical setting appropriate.

R

registered nurse a professional qualified by education and authorized by law to practice nursing. The professional nurse who works with the elderly combines basic nursing knowledge and skills with specialized knowledge of aging.

rehabilitation the use of medical, social, educational, and vocational therapy to return those **disabled** or otherwise incapacitated by **illness** or injury to an acceptable level of functional ability.

rehabilitation hospital an institution which provides **rehabilitation** services, usually physical rehabilitation, but also rehabilitation from alcohol or **substance abuse,** or from other disabling conditions.

rehabilitation unit a designated section of a hospital or other healthcare facility which provides **rehabilitation** services on either an inpatient or outpatient basis.

residential care facility: see **personal care service.**

resource utilization groups (RUGs) classification system which uses diagnostic information and **activities of daily living** to establish payments to **long term care** facilities under the **Medicaid** system. This system currently is being used in the state of New York and is being tested in other states.

respite care infrequent and temporary substitute care or supervision of a frail or disabled person, in the absence of the usual caregiver, or to provide relief for the normal caregiver. Respite services can be provided in home and out of home through a variety of resources including individuals, inpatient facilities, home health agencies, and **adult day care programs.**

rest home: see **personal care service.**

retirement village a form of community housing designed to meet the special needs of elderly retired persons. In addition to **independent housing** quarters, a retirement village may provide some combination of medical, nonmedical, and **personal care services.** Ideally, it will include, or at least provide for referral to, an **intermediate care facility, skilled nursing facility,** and **nursing home.** See also **life care community.**

S

screening clinic a diagnostic facility or service in which persons are tested for one or more specific conditions (e.g., hypertension, sickle cell anemia, respiratory ailments).

senior apartments: see **housing (elderly).**

senior citizen center a facility where older persons can participate in social, physical, health, and educational activities to support their health maintenance, independence, and involvement in the community.

senior citizen subscription program any of a number of programs for older persons in which subscribers, for a small annual fee, receive a package of basic benefits (e.g., membership in a **health promotion** program, a newsletter, **referral services,** and discounted meals e.g.,in a hospital cafeteria). In addition, individual programs can offer supplementary benefits such as pharmacy discounts. Subscribers are also given financial incentives to use the institution which sponsors the subscription program. CareLink is an example of such a program. Begun by the Sisters of St. Joseph Health System, Nazareth, MI, it offers services through some 31 hospitals in 5 states, for 40,000 subscribers. Mercy 65 is a senior citizens' assistance program offered by Catholic Healthcare West, Burlingame, CA.

service management: see **care management.**

signatory a term used to indicate the person who puts down a name at the end of an instrument to attest its validity or to signify consent. The "signature" may be made either by the person named or by delegating the authority to write or make the signature or by adopting one written or made for him/her. For example, one may grant power of attorney to another delegating authority to sign certain documents.

skilled nursing facility (SNF) under **Medicare** and **Medicaid,** an institution (or a distinct part of an institution) which has in effect a transfer agreement with one or more participating hospitals, and which is primarily engaged in providing skilled nursing care and related services for patients requiring medical or **nursing care** or **rehabilitation** services for injured, disabled, or sick persons; has formal policies developed with the advice of a group of professionals, including one or more **physicians** and **registered nurses,** to oversee the skilled nursing care and related medical or other services provided; has a physician, a registered nurse, or a medical staff responsible for the execution of such policies; requires that the healthcare of every patient be supervised by a physician, and provides for having a physician available to furnish necessary medical care in case of an emergency; maintains medical records on all patients; provides 24-hour nursing service and has at least one full-time registered nurse; provides appropriate methods and procedures for the dispensing and administering of drugs and biologicals; has a utilization review plan which meets legal requirements; is duly licensed, where this is required, or otherwise approved by the appropriate agency; has an overall plan and budget, including an operating budget and a 3-year capital expenditure plan; and meets other requirements related to the ownership of the facility, independent medical review of patients, provisions of the Life Safety Code and other applicable fire and safety codes and is managed by a licensed **nursing home** administrator.

social health maintenance organization a system of care for the elderly in which a single provider organization assumes responsibility for a full range of ambulatory, **acute** inpatient, **rehabilitative, nursing home,** and **personal care services** under a prospectively determined fixed budget. This model of comprehensive care for the elderly was developed by the University Health Policy Consortium at Brandeis University, under a planning grant awarded in 1980 by the Health Care Financing Administration. It is being implemented in four demonstration sites by the following organizations: The Metropolitan Jewish Geriatric Center (Brooklyn, NY); Kaiser Permanente Medical Care Program (Portland, OR); Ebenezer Society (Minneapolis, MN); and Senior Care Action Program (Long Beach, CA).

The major innovative features of the model are:

- comprehensive health and **long term care** (LTC) benefits
- consolidation of health and LTC under **care management** in one organized delivery system
- a provider organization being at financial risk for both medical care and LTC
- voluntary enrollment of an elderly population with a broad spectrum of healthcare needs from well to severely disabled
- active participation of both **Medicaid** and non-Medicaid-eligible **Medicare** enrollees
- pooled private and public financing of health and LTC services
- extension of **insurance** principles to LTC

social service professional counseling, provision of information, referral for service, or coordination of a client's relationships with family and community. Referral may be to such services as financial advice, legal aid, job assistance, housing assistance, or family counseling.

social work services provided by professionally trained social workers to enable a patient, family members, or others to deal with problems of social functioning affecting the patient's **health** or well-being.

speech therapy the study, examination, evaluation, and treatment of defects and **diseases** of the voice, of speech, and of spoken and written language, as well as the use of appropriate substitutional devices and treatment.

spend down a method whereby an individual reduces his/her gross income by incurring medical expenses until net income (after medical expenses) is low enough to meet a specified standard of need and thus to make the preson eligible for a medical care program. The spend down is equivalently a sliding scale deductible related to the individual's income level. For example, if eligibility requires that a person have a monthly income of $300 or less, a person with a $400 income would be covered after spending $100 out-of-pocket on medical care; one with an income of $450 would be covered only after out-of-pocket medical expenses of $150.

The term spend down originated in the **Medicaid** program; an individual whose income makes him/her ineligible for welfare, but is insufficient to pay for medical care, can become Medicaid-eligible as a medically needy person by spending some income on medical care. Eligibility requirements may also influence persons to divest themselves of assets.

sub-acute medical intervention a program of care specifically designed to intervene in the course of an illness beyond the **acute care** phase. This care incorporates a multidisciplinary approach to an individual's medical and emotional state that aggressively promotes therapy and medical treatment under medical staff direction and supervision. All treatment modalities are oriented toward restoration of the individual's highest attainable level of **health.** On the continuum of sub-acute medical intervention, an integral program objective is patient/family education.

substance abuse a generic term for the persistent or sporadic use of alcohol or drugs, inconsistent with or unrelated to acceptable medical or cultural practice. See also **alcoholism, drug dependence.**

supportive care room, board, and other **personal care services** generally provided on a long-term basis, which do not include a medical component. Such services are generally not covered by private or public **health insurance** or medical care programs, except as incidental to inpatient medical care in a hospital or nursing home. Custodial care may, however, be covered by **catastrophic** or **long term care health insurance.**

swing bed a bed designated by a public authority to be used interchangeably as a **long term care** bed or an **acute care** bed, depending on the care needs of an institution's current patient population.

T

team group of professionals working together in the care of the frail older adult in order to maximize the functional abilities of that person. Core team includes **physician,** nurse, and social worker; other usually essential team members are occupational and physical therapists and nutritionists; other important potential team members include pharmacists, dentists, opthamologists, podiatrists, and audiologists, etc.

telephone reassurance a telephone encounter with a person for the purpose of reducing social isolation, assuring **health** and safety, determining if special assistance is required, providing psychological reassurance, or notifying a contact person if the person called does not answer.

transportation service organized service to convey an individual from one location to another for an identified service population of the elderly or handicapped.

V

visiting nurse association (VNA) a voluntary organization that provides a variety of **home healthcare** services, using nurses and other trained personnel. Services include **nursing care; health education,** supervision, and counseling; and bedside care. Visiting nurse associations have their origin in the home nursing agencies, such as the New York City Mission which provided care to the poor in the 1870s. The first VNAs were established in Buffalo, Boston, and Philadelphia in 1886–87.

W

wellness program any one of numerous programs designed to prevent disease or its consequences, to modify behavior and encourage more healthful habits, and to maintain good **health.** In addition to exercise classes and the like, designed to maintain physical fitness, wellness programs may include educational classes and workshops on diet, diagnosis of physical **illness,** psychological aid, self-administration of medication, and improvements in healthful living standards, and other aspects of health maintenance. See also **health education, health promotion, preventive medicine.**

APPENDIX B

Members of the CHA Task Force on Long Term Care Policy

Chairman
Most Rev. Joseph M. Sullivan, DD
Auxiliary Bishop of Brooklyn
Brooklyn, NY

Bro. Richard Daly, CSC
Executive Director
Texas Catholic Conference
Austin, TX

Rev. Msgr. Charles J. Fahey
Director
Third Age Center
New York, NY

Sr. M. Caritas Geary, SP
President
Mercy Hospital
Springfield, MA

Claus Hamann, MD
Director of Geriatric Medicine
St. Francis Hospital and Medical Center
Hartford, CT

Most Rev. Oscar Lipscomb, DD
Archbishop of Mobile
Mobile, AL

Ellen McKay
Coordinator on Aging
Diocese of Lansing
Lansing, MI

Gary Ross
Center of Gerontology
St. Joseph Health System
Flint, MI

David Ward
Senior Vice President/Geriatrics
Catholic Health Corporation
Omaha, NE

Sr. Mary Eileen Wilhelm, RSM
Administrator/CEO
Mercy Medical
Daphne, AL

Ex Officio
John E. Curley, Jr.
President
CHA

Staff
William J. Cox
Vice President
CHA Division of Government Services

Joanne Elden
Government Liaison
CHA Division of Government Services

Sr. Elizabeth McMillan, RSM, PhD
Senior Associate
CHA Division of Theology, Mission, and Ethics

Lawrence Seidl
Senior Associate
CHA Division of Theology, Mission, and Ethics

Lola J. Westhoff
Senior Associate
CHA Division of Member Services

Special Observers
Bro. Joseph Berg, CSC
Catholic Charities USA
Washington, DC

Sharon Daly
United States Catholic Conference
Washington, DC

Sr. Suzanne E. Sattler, IHM
Sisters of Mercy Health Corporation
Farmington Hills, MI

APPENDIX C

Presenters to the Task Force on Long Term Care Policy

Sr. Rose Teresa Bahr, ASC
Center on Aging
The Catholic University of America
Washington, DC

Daniel Callahan, PhD
The Hastings Center
Hastings-on-Hudson, NY

Bartholomew J. Callopy, PhD
The Hastings Center
Hastings-on-Hudson, NY

Jack Guralnick
National Institute on Aging
Bethesda, MD

Sr. Margaret Rose Whiteneck, CBS
Bon Secours Hospital—Villa Marie Nursing Center
North Miami, FL

Robert Wildenhaus
The DePaul/Mount St. Vincent and St. Joseph Residence
Seattle, WA

APPENDIX D

Outsider Reviewers of the Task Force Report

James J. McCormack, PhD
Fordham University
New York, NY

Sr. Margaret Rose Whiteneck, CBS
Bon Secours Hospital—Villa Marie Nursing Center
North Miami, FL

Mathew H. Ahmann
Catholic Charities USA
Washington, DC

APPENDIX E

Bibliography

For Additional Reading
on the Continuum of Care and Issues
Affecting the Elderly-at-Risk

1. *Managing the Continuum of Care,* ed. Connie J. Evashwick and Lawrence J. Weiss, Aspen Publishers, Inc., Rockville, MD, 1987.
2. Kevin D. O'Rourke, *Development of Church Teaching on Prolonging Life,* The Catholic Health Association of the United States, St. Louis, 1988.
3. Marvin Wilensky, "Pressure Increases for Development of a National Long-Term Care Policy," *Federation of American Health Systems Review,* January-February 1988, pp. 36-38.
4. Marvin Wilensky, "In Focus," *The Aging Connection,* February-March 1988, pp. 9-10.
5. Barbara Waxman, "Case Management for Older Adults," *Optimal Health,* January-February 1988, pp. 22-24.
6. Pat Wahlstedt and Wanda Balser, "The Long Term Care Continuum," *The Kansas Nurse,* November 1984, pp. 3-5.
7. Pat Wahlstedt and Wanda Balser, "Multihospital Systems Target Continuum of Care Strategy," *Hospitals,* March 1, 1985, pp. 52, 56-57.
8. Stanley J. Brody, "Continuum of Care: The New-Old Health Requirement," *Michigan Hospitals,* October 1986, pp. 17-21.
9. William A. Read and James C. O'Brien, "New Trends in Hospital-Based Services for the Elderly," *Trustee,* September 1986, pp. 20-22.
10. "Medicare: Coming of Age. A Proposal for Reform," Center for Health Policy and Management, John F. Kennedy School of Government, Harvard University, Cambridge, MA, 1986.
11. Sr. Margaret Rose Whiteneck, CBS, "Forum Allows LTC Facilities to Face Ethical Issues Together," *Health Progress,* January-February 1988, pp. 82-84.
12. Msgr. Charles J. Fahey, "Challenges of Long-Term Care Call for New Policies," *Health Progress,* January-February 1988, pp. 38-40, 47.
13. Sr. M. Frances Schumer, ASC, and Connie March, RN, "Creating a Quality Assurance Program for Long-Term Care," *Health Progress,* November 1987.
14. Barbara Cox and Lois Waller, *Communicating with the Elderly,* The Catholic Health Association of the United States, St. Louis, 1987.
15. Alice M. Rivlin and Joshua M. Wiener, *Caring for the Disabled Elderly: Who Will Pay?* The Brookings Institution, Washington, DC, 1988.
16. *No Room in the Marketplace: The Health Care of the Poor,* The Catholic Health Association of the United States, St. Louis, 1986.

Continuum of Care Models

St. Camillus Health and Rehabilitation Center/Mahan Gorham Manor Syracuse, NY

In the 1930s, the pastor of St. Patrick's Church in Jordan, NY acquired a house and the vacant land next to it in Albridge, NY, with the intent of building a new parish church and using the house as a rectory. The plans for a new church in the rural area never materialized, but the house itself continued to be minimally heated and maintained. Six years ago, the current pastor approached Catholic Charities of the Diocese of Syracuse regarding other possible uses for the property. With the sponsorship of St. Camillus Health and Rehabilitation Center, Catholic Charities undertook the renovation of the house for an "Enriched Housing Program" for the community. Catholic Charities raised $200,000 from government, community, and private sources for building, renovating, and providing appliances for the house, with the hope of providing a noninstitutional living setting for six elderly persons.

In 1986, Catholic Charities turned over the management to St. Camillus and Mahan Gorham Manor opened with six residents. Five of the original residents are still there, and the current number of residents is seven. All the residents are female, and require some degree of help with independent living. Three original participants were referred to the program directly from St. Camillus, where they had been residents. The others were referred from the community. Several residents attend adult day care and occupational and speech therapy at St. Camillus, 15 miles away. Without the "Enriched Housing Program," all would be at risk of institutionalization. The program is governed by Albridge Adult Community, Inc., a voluntary, not-for-profit organization. Each resident has a private room and all the residents are over 65 years of age. The monthly charge of $650 is paid for by the residents themselves, all of whom receive either private pensions or SSI. The program is designed to be financially self-sustaining. The program employs a part-time cook and part-time handyman, as well as a social worker and director. A full-time manager lives in the house.

The community provides broad support and enthusiasm for the program, offering gifts of food and transportation to the residents. Once a month, the residents enjoy going out for dinner to a local restaurant. The "Enriched Housing Program" has also been featured on CBS "On the Road with Charles Kuralt."

St. Joseph Health Systems, Inc.
Flint, Michigan

St. Joseph Health Systems, Flint, MI, was established in 1980 by St. Joseph Hospital as a hospital-based health system. It has rapidly expanded to develop a continuum of health related services encompassing not only in-patient and out-patient acute care, but also an extensive network of extended and home-based care services.

As a nonprofit holding company, St. Joseph Health Systems is comprised of 20 subsidiary corporations including 4 acute care facilities with over 900 licensed beds, a licensed 140-bed skilled nursing facility, an adult day care program, primary care out-patient health centers, a home health agency, a certified hospice, a private-duty nursing service, a durable medical equipment company, a commercial laboratory company, and a center for gerontology which includes geriatric care management.

Serving a three-county geographic area, St. Joseph Health Systems was developed by St. Joseph Hospital as part of a strategic plan to strengthen and solidify its market position and better meet the changing healthcare needs of the community. After conducting an environmental assessment and reaffirming that its mission is healthcare and not just acute care, St. Joseph Hospital concluded that it was in an excellent position to develop and coordinate a comprehensive system of services, especially those needed by the older population.

An important component of St. Joseph Health Systems is its linkage with other community agencies. Consequently, many of the subsidiaries of St. Joseph Health Systems were existing providers in the St. Joseph's service area before they became part of the system. Other subsidiary services were developed in response to assessments of community need taking into account potential financing and regulatory constraints, competition, and opportunities for collaboration.

Essential to its continuum of care strategy, St. Joseph Health Systems has consistently moved to establish a client-focused system of care. Crucial to the success of the continuum is its ability to coordinate client usage of a comprehensive array of health and social services spanning all levels of intensity. To this end, St. Joseph Health Systems is attempting to put in place a number of integrating mechanisms to insure a cost-effective, coordinated system of services for its clients.

The geriatric care management program operated through the Center for Gerontology provides one of the key integrating mechanisms for insuring that patients who have complex multiple problems receive the services they require. It provides a support system for patients by selecting services as needed from those offered within the health services continuum. It also has established referral and service agreements with over 50 agencies outside St. Joseph Health Systems. By providing care coordination for complex cases, it is a service which promotes cost containment and preserves quality by tracking and monitoring clients' service usage.

On the management information side, St. Joseph Health Systems does not as yet have a computer system in place that can access and integrate data from all the services in the continuum. However, some subsidiaries have moved to integrate their data systems with that of one of the hospitals, enabling them to track patients as they move from one type of service to another. A long-term goal of the health system is to establish a central registration process and tracking system that will allow each client's progress to be monitored and will integrate the client's health, social, and financial data.

By developing its continuum of care, St. Joseph Health Systems is strengthening its financial position by generating savings from economies of scale, efficiencies of operation, increased marketshare and revenues from new lines of business, and an ability to respond to managed care and capitated payment systems.

The Catholic Health Association of the United States is the national organization of Catholic hospitals and long term care facilities, their sponsoring organizations and systems, and other health and related agencies and services operated as Catholic. It is an ecclesial community participating in the mission of the Catholic Church through its members' ministry of healing. CHA witnesses this ministry by providing leadership both within the Church and within the broader society and through its programs of education, facilitation, and advocacy.

This document represents one more service of The Catholic Health Association of the United States, 4455 Woodson Road, St. Louis, MO 63134-0889, 314-427-2500.